Financial Management in Health Services

Understanding Public Health

Series editors: Nick Black and Rosalind Raine, London School of Hygiene & Tropical Medicine

Throughout the world, recognition of the importance of public health to sustainable, safe and healthy societies is growing. The achievements of public health in nineteenth-century Europe were for much of the twentieth century overshadowed by advances in personal care, in particular in hospital care. Now, with the dawning of a new century, there is increasing understanding of the inevitable limits of individual health care and of the need to complement such services with effective public health strategies. Major improvements in people's health will come from controlling communicable diseases, eradicating environmental hazards, improving people's diets and enhancing the availability and quality of effective health care. To achieve this, every country needs a cadre of knowledgeable public health practitioners with social, political and organizational skills to lead and bring about changes at international, national and local levels.

This is one of a series of 20 books that provides a foundation for those wishing to join in and contribute to the twenty-first-century regeneration of public health, helping to put the concerns and perspectives of public health at the heart of policy-making and service provision. While each book stands alone, together they provide a comprehensive account of the three main aims of public health: protecting the public from environmental hazards, improving the health of the public and ensuring high quality health services are available to all. Some of the books focus on methods, others on key topics. They have been written by staff at the London School of Hygiene & Tropical Medicine with considerable experience of teaching public health to students from low, middle and high income countries. Much of the material has been developed and tested with postgraduate students both in face-to-face teaching and through distance learning.

The books are designed for self-directed learning. Each chapter has explicit learning objectives, key terms are highlighted and the text contains many activities to enable the reader to test their own understanding of the ideas and material covered. Written in a clear and accessible style, the series will be essential reading for students taking postgraduate courses in public health and will also be of interest to public health practitioners and policy-makers.

Titles in the series

Analytical models for decision making: Colin Sanderson and Reinhold Gruen
Controlling communicable disease: Norman Noah
Economic analysis for management and policy: Stephen Jan, Lilani Kumaranayake,
    Jenny Roberts, Kara Hanson and Kate Archibald
Economic evaluation: Julia Fox-Rushby and John Cairns (eds)
Environmental epidemiology: Paul Wilkinson (ed)
Environment, health and sustainable development: Megan Landon
Environmental health policy: David Ball
Financial management in health services: Reinhold Gruen and Anne Howarth
Global change and health: Kelley Lee and Jeff Collin (eds)
Health care evaluation: Sarah Smith, Don Sinclair, Rosalind Raine and Barnaby Reeves
Health promotion practice: Maggie Davies, Wendy Macdowall and Chris Bonell (eds)
Health promotion theory: Maggie Davies and Wendy Macdowall (eds)
Introduction to epidemiology: Lucianne Bailey, Katerina Vardulaki, Julia Langham and
    Daniel Chandramohan
Introduction to health economics: David Wonderling, Reinhold Gruen and Nick Black
Issues in public health: Joceline Pomerleau and Martin McKee (eds)
Making health policy: Kent Buse, Nicholas Mays and Gill Walt
Managing health services: Nick Goodwin, Reinhold Gruen and Valerie Iles
Medical anthropology: Robert Pool and Wenzel Geissler
Principles of social research: Judith Green and John Browne (eds)
Understanding health services: Nick Black and Reinhold Gruen

Financial Management in Health Services

Reinhold Gruen and Anne Howarth

Open University Press

Open University Press
McGraw-Hill Education
McGraw-Hill House
Shoppenhangers Road
Maidenhead
Berkshire
England
SL6 2QL

email: enquiries@openup.co.uk
world wide web: www.openup.co.uk

and Two Penn Plaza, New York, NY 10121-2289, USA

First published 2005

A catalogue record of this book is available from the British Library

ISBN-10: 0 335 218512
ISBN-13: 978 0 335 218516

Library of Congress Cataloging-in-Publication Data
CIP data has been applied for

Typeset by RefineCatch Limited, Bungay, Suffolk
Printed in Poland by OZGraf. S.A.
www.polskabook.pl

Contents

Acknowledgements

Open University Press and the London School of Hygiene and Tropical Medicine have made every effort to obtain permission from copyright holders to reproduce material in this book and to acknowledge these sources correctly. Any omissions brought to our attention will be remedied in future editions.

We would like to express our grateful thanks to the following copyright holders for granting permission to reproduce material in this book.

p. 15	Adapted from Barnum, H., Kutzin, J. and Saxenian, H. (1995) 'Incentives and provider payment methods', HRO Working Paper No.51. Washington DC, World Bank.
p. 15	Adapted from Donaldson, C. and Gerard, K. (1992) Economics of Health Care Financing: The Visible Hand. London: Macmillan 1992.
p. 210	Figure 6.8, page 92 from Mellett H, Marriott N and Harries S, Financial Management in the NHS:A Manager's Handbook, Thomson Learning, 1993 by permission of Thomson Learning.
p. 67–8	Based on "Charging Fees for Family Planning Services", The Family Planning Manager, vol. 1, no. 3, 1992. Used with permission from Management Sciences for Health, Cambridge, Massachusetts.

Overview of the book

Introduction

This book is intended to help you to develop your financial skills and learn how to manage money as effectively as you manage people or services, or make clinical decisions. You need financial management skills to help ensure that you make the right decisions so that you use the money you have to its best effect. And if you can do this, you are contributing to something much bigger – getting better health care to more people. This is what financial management in health services is about. This book will not turn you into a financial expert able to produce vast quantities of numbers and statistics. Neither will it make you able to produce a set of accounts in double-quick time. But it will show you how to find your way around a set of accounts, or your budget, or the financial projections for a new service development, and how to examine these incisively, spot the key issues and discuss these confidently with financial experts and senior management.

A benefit of reading this book is a much better understanding of your own organization's financial performance and of its accounting system. To achieve this, however, you must be prepared to seek out relevant information from your finance department, asking questions of your finance colleagues and obtaining copies of your own organization's financial statements.

You may find that financial statements in your country look different from what is presented in this book. This may be due to differences in the terminology used, in which case you would need to translate terms used here into the equivalent terms used in your country. Or you may find that financial statements are very basic or incomplete, as financial reporting systems are still being developed, as is the case in many low- and middle-income countries. You may also find that accounts and budgets are not available at your level of the organization because financial responsibility is not devolved to that level. The book takes account of this as it starts with the basic concepts of costing and goes on via management accounting to the more complex areas of financial reporting and governance.

Why study financial management?

You may have studied financial management as part of a management course or you may have experience of financial management and therefore have a very good idea about the role of financial management in health services. But you may not have had a chance to see the bigger picture – how what you do fits into the overall financial management of the organization. Studying financial management will help.

Even if you are not working in an environment which produces sophisticated financial statements, a basic understanding of financial accounts will help you enter discussions with financial managers or to work on the supervisory board of a health care organization and ask the right questions about its financial performance.

Structure of the book

Each chapter includes:

- an overview;
- learning objectives;
- key terms;
- a range of activities;
- feedback to or other discussion around the activities;
- a summary.

To get the most out of this book you will need to obtain the following information:

- the ways health services in your country are financed (Chapter 1);
- the budget of your organization (Chapters 2 and 7);
- the latest set of accounts for your organization (Chapters 1, 8, 10–14) (alternatively you can use the accounts provided in Appendix 1).

You will need a calculator for some of the activities or, alternatively, you may wish to set up simple computer spreadsheets.

The book consists of four sections.

Introduction

You will first, in Chapter 1, be introduced to the context of financial management in health care: the different ways of funding health services and of paying providers of health services as well as the reasons for rising health care expenditure and efforts to control costs. In Chapter 2 you will learn about the main areas of responsibility of the finance department and why an understanding of financial management is essential to all managers in any organization.

Management accounting

You will then go on, in Chapters 3 to 8, to learn how management accounting techniques can help you as a manager to analyse the costs incurred by your department, to ensure that the charges made are adequate to cover the costs of the services provided and to use budgets to plan and control the activities of your unit.

Financial accounting

Chapter 9 introduces financial accounting and the concepts on which it is based. In Chapters 10 to 12 the three principal accounting statements are introduced and you will have the opportunity to undertake a guided analysis of each of these statements for your own organization and for a large hospital. Chapters 13 and 14 review the management of working capital and financial analysis, areas of financial accounting that are particularly relevant to all managers.

Financial control and information systems

In Chapters 15 to 17 you will explore accounting systems and financial and regulatory controls. In Chapters 18 and 19 you will focus on information for decision-making, including performance management and information to assist in making capital investment decisions. Finally, in Chapter 20, you will learn about financial aspects of project management.

Acknowledgements

The authors acknowledge the contribution of: Greg Layther in developing an earlier version on which the content of several chapters is based; David King, Assistant Director of Investment at North East London Strategic Health Authority, for detailed comments and advice on the book; and Deirdre Byrne (series manager) for help and support.

SECTION I

Introduction

Introduction to financial management

Overview

It is important that health services managers make the best possible use of the resources available to them. Whatever your area of management responsibility, financial management skills enable you to use financial information to ensure that you do so. In this chapter you will be introduced to the context of financial management, particularly the basic principles of financing health care and paying providers, as well as the institutional contexts in which health services operate.

Learning objectives

By the end of this chapter you should be able to:

- **outline the different ways of funding health services**
- **understand the different ways of paying providers of health services**
- **analyse ways of regulating the private/public mix, both in finance and in provision of health services**
- **outline the principles of new public sector management and their implications for financial reforms of the public health sector**

Key terms

Beveridge system A health system funded through public revenue raised by general taxation, named after Sir William Beveridge.

Bismarck system A health system funded through payroll-based social insurance contributions, named after Otto von Bismarck.

Co-payments (user fees) Direct payments made by users of health services as a contribution to their cost (eg prescription charges)

Financial management Managerial activities of obtaining and disbursing funds, financial planning, reporting and risk management.

New public management An approach to government involving the application of private sector management techniques.

Outcomes Change in status as a result of the system processes (in health services context, the change in health status as a result of care).

Private/public mix The mix of public and private funders and providers of health services.

Provider payment methods The different ways of paying health care providers such as fee for service, capitation and case base reimbursement.

> **Residual claimant status** The arrangements under which a person or agency – the residual claimant – is entitled to retain an organization's surplus or is held responsible to bear its financial loss.

What is financial management?

For many people, financial management may seem a complex and mysterious activity which is best left to the finance department. However, over the last few decades an understanding of financial management has become important not only to accountants but also to health professionals and clinical managers.

Managers are involved in a range of operational and strategic decisions in which financial issues play a key role. This could be simple questions such as:

* How would a 3 per cent pay rise for nurses affect the budget?

Or more complex problems such as:

* Would we be able to expand mother and child health service activity by 10 per cent with the funds available?
* At which level should user fees be set?
* Can we afford to open a new trauma department and hire the required staff?
* Are our funds sufficient to cover vaccinating all children in our district?
* What is the rate of return on the capital investment of equipping and building a new health centre?
* Why has the health centre incurred a loss of $500,000 and what measures should be taken to improve financial performance in the next year?

Health care managers have continuously to respond to challenges related to financial management. You will find that there are many decisions such as decentralizing or centralizing health services, and decisions on privatization, mergers or acquisition of health care organizations. All these decisions require input from both the financial department and from other areas of expertise. Thus, financial management impinges on all aspects of the organization and is integrated with all other managerial activities to achieve the overall strategic goals of the organization.

Financial management is important to keep the organization going and to ensure that resources are used in the best possible way; it entails a range of activities related to obtaining and disbursing funds, financial planning, reporting and risk management. This general definition covers both the macro level of a health system and the meso level of an organization. However, financial information should not be seen as isolated from the rest of the organization. The understanding of financial information requires interdisciplinary knowledge of how health services operate and how management decisions are influenced by their political, economic and organizational environment. Thus the financial system can be seen as an essential subsystem of the health system. This relationship becomes clearer if you look at the basic model underlying health care which can be described in terms of:

input → process → outcomes

Each of these elements has a financial dimension:

- *Input* means the resources which are used to produce health care. These are, for example, staff, assets, facilities, equipment and consumables. All these inputs can be measured and valued in a common expression – money. Thus monetary values of the inputs are the common language which allows resource use to be analysed within a single or across several organizations.
- *Process* describes the various activities (employing inputs) so that the desired outcome is achieved. Financial processes involve collecting revenue, paying staff and customers, buying drugs and medical supplies, and investing capital in buildings and equipment. To be able to perform these operations in a meaningful way, the financial information used needs to be accurate, timely and relevant. Examples of health care processes are the number of X-rays, operations, vaccinations, bed days or cases of patients treated.
- *Outcomes* measure the changes to a patient's health status that can be attributed to the preceding health care and therefore implicitly to the financial resources consumed. Outcome measures, such as quality of life or survival, play an important role in economic evaluation – for example, assessing the inputs required to produce one additional healthy life year or a defined increase in quality of life.

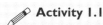 **Activity 1.1**

1 Identify the types of resources used by the organization for which you work. Note that a distinction can be made between human and material resources. Material resources can be subdivided into *capital items* that have a life span longer than one year (land, buildings, equipment), and *recurrent* or *revenue items* that are consumed in less than one year (medical supplies, consumables, energy supply).
2 For the organization for which you work, give examples of possible measures of processes and outcomes.

 Feedback

1 The range of resources used by your organization will encompass staff, all assets, such as land and buildings, equipment, supplies and consumables that are needed to produce the service. If working in a TB unit, you would list staff, microscopes and laboratory equipment, vehicles for specimen transport, and drugs and facilities for treating patients. The common basis of comparing resources is the monetary value attached to each item of input.

2 Health care organizations use a range of measures of processes. In the case of the TB unit, these would be the number of cases detected or the number of patients treated. Measuring outcome would take account of the benefits provided by the treatment, for example, the cure rate and patient satisfaction with treatment. You could work out the financial resources consumed per case detected or patient cured.

Health care finance

Decisions in financial management are largely shaped by the economic, political, social and legal environment in which the organization operates. Availability and use of financial resources in health care are influenced by the following three dimensions:

- the method of financing health care;
- the methods of provider payment;
- the institutional context in which the health care organization operates.

One of the key functions of financial management is the acquisition of funds, so it is worthwhile thinking how the income of the organization is generated. If you take a societal viewpoint, ultimately all money that is spent on health care originates from private households, thus the fundamental financial transaction is the conversion of household income into provider income. As shown in Figure 1.1 there are two basic ways of paying for health care.

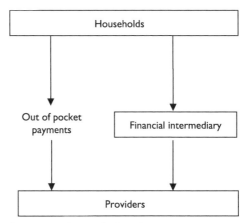

Figure 1.1 The two basic ways of paying for health care

Out of pocket payment is still a frequent and common form of paying for health care. But, because of the uncertainty of need and potentially high costs of care, third-party payment by government or insurance company is a preferred alternative. This means that a *financial intermediary* is involved in the transaction between households and providers. Households pay taxes or premiums entitling them to access to care. Providers receive payment from the financial intermediary and may have to deal with different sources of funds. Despite coverage by insurance or government, patients may be charged co-payments and user fees to control demand or to raise additional revenue for the health sector.

While internationally, sources of funding vary widely, three different models of health care financing systems can be distinguished according to the prevailing type of financial intermediary:

1 *Tax-based systems (Beveridge systems)* are mainly funded through public revenue, raised by general taxation. Government may act as financial agent and as

provider of health services. Equity of financing is achieved by progressive taxation. Providers receive direct funds from government which cover all basic health care spending, so that services are free at the point of use. Health care expenditure is planned centrally and allocated according to need to decentralized provider units, thus ensuring equity of access to health care. Examples include the Spanish National Health Service and many health systems in Africa, Southern and Eastern Europe, and South Asia.

2 *Social health insurance (Bismarck systems)* are based on compulsory contributions entitling the insured persons and their families to a defined range of health services. Social insurance companies normally do not act as providers. Financial resources are earmarked for health and equity of financing is achieved by progressive tariffs and policies which include coverage for family members and children. Financial resources follow the individual patient, thus ensuring equity of access for all insured persons. Services are free at the point of use and providers bill the insurance company for the individual patient treated. Examples include countries in Western Europe, Latin America and South-East Asia.

3 *Private health insurance* is based on actuarially determined premiums and voluntary enrolment by individuals or employers. Insurance schemes may differ widely with respect to reimbursement levels and choice of providers. Increasingly, managed care schemes are used that give access to defined packages of care and restrict patient choice to networks of selected providers. In contrast to the other systems, private health insurance is not effective in achieving universal coverage – that is, insuring the entire population of a country. The USA is one of the few countries that depends on private insurance as a major source of funding for health care. In most countries, private insurance plays only a complementary or even a marginal role.

External aid

In many low-income countries, external aid is a substantial source of funding. External aid usually takes the form of loans or grants. It can make up between 20 and 90 per cent of the total public health expenditure (WHO 1995). The main approaches to financing are project aid, programme aid and sector aid (Cassels 1997):

- *Project aid* provides financial resources for a time-limited discrete activity in the health sector – for example, building a new hospital.
- *Programme aid* describes a variety of forms of long-term external aid which usually takes the form of budget support. A distinction can be made between vertical and horizontal programmes:
  - Vertical programmes are characterized by funds focusing on specific diseases such as HIV-Aids, TB or polio. Many of the vertical programmes are funded by the multilateral aid agencies such as the World Health Organization (WHO) and the World Bank and run at national level with an independent financial management structure.
  - Horizontal programmes aim to support the main health services infrastructure – for example, strengthening the provision of primary health services in a region. Financial support is aimed at all facilities of the same level of care in a region and financial management is part of the main organization structure.

- *Health sector aid* integrates all forms of financial aid into a single, comprehensive approach to financial management. It is not a specific form of aid, like project or programme aid. Rather, it reflects a shift in policy, based on the notion that the joint effort of the donor community is more effective than isolated activities of different donors. Donor consortia are formed in order to work together with the recipient government on an overall strategy and a consistent basis for financial planning for the entire health sector. The aim is to integrate separated areas of service delivery and to channel all funds from donors into general budget support (Briggs *et al.* 2002).

None of the different forms of aid in itself guarantees a sustainable and affordable means of finance. To reduce dependency from external aid, it is increasingly used to finance start-up costs and the development of infrastructure. In addition there is a stronger focus on mobilizing additional resources for the health sector. User fees and prepaid schemes or basic forms of health insurance have been introduced on a larger scale in order to raise additional revenue and improve the quality of service provision.

Flow of funds in health care

Considering the large range of sources and uses of funds, both government and organizations need reliable financial information to assess the flow of funds, assess past performance and make plans for the future. There are two principal approaches to financial reporting: *accounts* inform on past expenditure and *budgets* are financial plans for the future.

A way of looking at the flow of funds at the macro level is to analyse national health accounts (NHAs). NHAs have attracted attention in recent years because they give an overview of all sources and uses of health care funds in a country. The accounts present financial information which is usually subdivided into various categories as shown in Table 1.1. Thus NHAs give a comprehensive picture of private and public health care spending in a country and are an important tool of planning.

Table 1.1 The categories in a national health account

	Category	*Examples*
Sources	Private/public financial agents	Households, government, social health insurance, private health insurance, external aid
Uses	Form of payment	Premium, taxation, out of pocket
	Providers	Hospitals, health centres
	Functions	Inpatient, outpatient, primary, secondary, tertiary care
	Line items	Salaries, drugs, equipment
	Geographic	Urban – rural
	Socioeconomic	Social class, ethnic group, income levels, insured/uninsured population

✐ Activity 1.2

This activity asks you to reflect on the ways health care providers obtain income for a sustainable service provision. For this activity you should try to get two pieces of information

a) From public sources (e.g. the Ministry of Health) the NHAs of your country or similar information regarding sources and uses of funds. You will also find information on NHAs on the WHO website.

b) From the financial department of your organization, your organization's annual financial report analysing and comparing sources and flows of funds.

1   What are the main sources of health care finance in your country?
2   What are the main sources of funding of your health care organization?
3   Take the main source of income and outline the flow of funds from the consumer to your organization.

↻ Feedback

1 Comparing NHAs across countries, some of the key evidence suggests that health care financing tends to be complex and relies on several sources. The distinction between Bismarck and Beveridge systems refers to the prevailing source of funding, either through social insurance or taxation. Usually there are several other forms of funding. Countries may rely on a mix of social and private insurance and taxation. In addition, in all countries there are varying levels of private health care spending. Many low-income countries rely also on external aid as a key source of finance.

2 The patterns of financing at national level may not completely translate into the patterns of income of health care organizations. However, many organizations will have at least two sources of income: government or insurance payments and direct payments from patients. In insurance-based systems, providers may have to deal with several purchasers of care. There may also be other forms of income, such as charitable donations, external aid, loans and grants. Funds from external aid may appear in a separate development budget or may be integrated with government funding.

3 Under social and private health insurance, households and employers pay contributions to the insurance companies which in turn reimburse providers for the service delivered to patients. In tax-funded systems, the Ministry of Finance is the central agency concerned with government's disbursement and collection systems for funds and provides central accounting and reporting for all public financial transactions. The agreed annual budget is administered by the Ministry of Health and disbursed to regional or district health authorities and from there to provider organizations.

Equity

A key concern in collecting funds and allocating resources is *equity*. Equity has at least two dimensions: *equity of finance* and *equity of use* of health care.

1   *Equity of finance* refers to a fair distribution of the financial burden, which is

usually achieved through progressive taxation or progressive tariffs for social insurance contributions.

2 *Equity of use* means equal treatment for equal needs, irrespective of ability to pay, age, sex, ethnicity, religion and geographic region.

In pursuing these goals, health systems may use a range of regulatory policies and economic incentives. In allocating resources across regions, some countries with public health systems use a formula based on population data in order to achieve equity in devolving central budgets to smaller geographic units (McPake *et al.* 2002). Elements of such a formula may include:

- demand factors such as
  - age, to reflect higher demand from infants and elderly people
  - mortality and morbidity, to reflect relative differences in health status between regions
  - socioeconomic factors affecting the need for services (household income, unemployment rates, elderly persons living alone);
- supply factors, such as regional cost differences in producing the service and the regional distribution of primary, secondary and tertiary care facilities.

The resource allocation process should allow for growth of the budget and deviation from historic spending patterns in order to direct funds to priority areas of need. In identifying priorities for funding, participation of key stakeholders can be helpful to facilitate data collection and to measure the achievement of equity objectives (Mbandwa *et al.* 2001).

Provider payment methods

Historically, provider payment methods have evolved along with the different forms of finance which have developed in a range of different ways:

1 *Fixed budgets* are most commonly used for allocating resources to health care providers and programmes. Overall expenditure can be controlled easily by defining limits for each spending category such as staff, equipment and medical supplies. While this approach is easy to administer, it is not very responsive to local needs. For example, funds that were not spent during the year may not be transferred to the next year or exchanged between spending categories. Increasingly, global budgets are used which give managers more flexibility. If necessary they can reallocate resources between spending categories and balance income and expenditure over more than one year. However, this approach requires good information about service costs and needs and a high level of discretion in managing staff, equipment and supplies. As a consequence, managers are entrusted with more accountability for the financial performance of the organization for which they are responsible. The introduction of devolved global budgets has been an important element in health sector reforms in many countries, particularly the decentralizing of health services.

2 *Capitation* is mainly used in primary care services and based on a fixed payment per insured person to cover for a defined package of services. This gives an incentive to reduce costs per case, but can also lead to selection of low-risk cases or inappropriate referrals.

3 *Fee-for-service (FFS)* involves each single item of service being paid for by the patient or third-party payer. If not combined with a budget cap, this may lead to

inappropriate provision of care, known as *supplier-induced demand*. Conversely, FFS can be used as an instrument to increase service provision in underserved areas of care.

4 *Case-based reimbursement* is based on an agreed sum (or tariff) which is paid for each category of patient or episode of care. In the hospital sector, this form of payment has largely replaced retrospective payment on the basis of bed days provided which generated incentives to increase length of stay. The methods of defining cases vary widely. Many countries use only a few categories such as distinguishing between inpatient and outpatient cases, or for the most common operations. The more complex methods are based on diagnosis-related groups (DRGs), which may consist of several hundred categories for reimbursement.

Each method affects provider behaviour in a specific way with different consequences for efficiency and quality of service provision. You may have noted that the term 'provider' refers both to individual health professionals as well as to organizations. At the organizational level, the motivational aspects of paying staff play an important role, though it is widely recognized that pay has its limitations as a motivator. Other non-financial incentives, such as career opportunities, status and social recognition may be equally important.

Financial management is mainly concerned with the institutional aspects of provider payment. The form these payments take influences the volume and quality of the services provided. Financial managers need to be aware of the consequences of the different payment methods in terms of:

- the economic incentives generated; and
- the ways the financial risk is distributed between the financial intermediary and the provider.

Table 1.2 shows potential incentives and disincentives and the distribution of risk in relation to different payment methods. The financial incentives set by the

Table 1.2 Potential incentives and distribution of risk associated with different provider payment methods

	Potential incentives to providers		Risk distribution
	Beneficial	Adverse	
Fixed budgets	Efficient service provision, cost reduction	Poor attention to quality	Shifts risk to provider
FFS	High attention to consumers, to expand care to underserved groups	Supplier-induced demand	High risk for financing agency, therefore fee regulation and global budgets needed
Capitation	To use cost-reducing technologies and effective treatments	Selection of low-risk cases, decrease in quantity of services per case	High risk for provider; additional provision for costly cases needed
Case-based, e.g. DRGs	Increases efficiency of care (compared to retrospective reimbursement)	'Dumping' of costly cases	Shifts risk to the provider; needs additional provisions to avoid adverse incentives.

Sources: Barnum *et al.* (1995); Donaldson and Gerard (1993)

payment method may be beneficial or adverse; this means they may have wanted or unwanted effects on the quality and volume of service provision. Financial risk relates to the question of who bears the costs caused by these effects if, for example, activity increases. For example, with FFS the financial risk rests with the purchaser while capitation shifts the risk to the provider. There is no single best payment method for health, and health systems use various ways to avoid the consequences of perverse incentives.

Activity 1.3

1 What are the main provider payment methods used in your country for primary and secondary care services?
2 What are the likely administrative requirements and costs associated with each method?

Feedback

1 Often a combination of methods is used to offset the disadvantages of any single method. There is a universal trend to use fixed budgets, which can be combined with any other payment method to contain overall costs.

2 Obviously the more complex payment methods are linked to relatively high administrative costs. Capitation is more expensive to manage than fixed budgets but less expensive than FFS and case-based reimbursement. You should be aware that some of the methods, such as case-based reimbursement, require well developed institutions and management skills. They may neither be feasible nor affordable in low-income countries.

Public/private mix of financing and provision of services

The organizational setting in which managers operate varies widely both internationally and within a country. Think of managers working in a:

- government-funded health centre;
- managed care company run by a private health insurance organization;
- non-governmental organization (NGO) hospital;
- vertical health programme, managed by the Ministry of Health.

The basic distinction you can make is between public and private sector organizations.

Public sector organizations can be responsible for both finance and provision of health services. They encompass not only government organizations at central, regional and local level but also public bodies with statutory responsibilities.

The *private sector* can be divided into for-profit and not-for-profit organizations. The former include, for example, the pharmaceutical industry and some hospitals or clinics, the latter the voluntary sector, charities and other NGOs pursuing humanitarian goals.

- *For-profit organizations* are owned by individuals or groups of shareholders and operate in areas of the health sector where they can make profits. They pay tax, can raise capital by issuing equity and they are expected to provide a return on the investments to the owners. The key motivator for their owners is making a profit but other aims not directly linked to returns may also apply, such as the market share and the company image.
- *Not-for-profit* private sector companies are owned by charities, mutual societies, health cooperatives or welfare organizations. They are usually exempted from tax as long as they reinvest any surplus made in the organization (including the remuneration of their staff). Many motives related to the mission of the organization play a role. They may use voluntary workers and may receive charitable donations and contributions as well as subsidies from government.

Activity 1.4

The public/private distinction refers both to financing and delivery of care. Use Figure 1.2 to assess the private/public mix in your country and find out where on the matrix primary care and hospital services would fit in terms of their financing and provision.

Provision of services

		Public	Private
Financing	Public	A	B
	Private	C	D

Figure 1.2 Assessing the private/public mix in health care

Feedback

Under A and D the situation is straightforward, with both finance and delivery of services being either public or private: examples are a government-owned hospital funded by social insurance (A) or a private practitioner paid out of pocket by their patients (D). Option B would apply, for example, to private practitioners who are paid out of public funds. Category C relates to private sources of financing in a public delivery context – for example, the capital injected into a public hospital under a private/public partnership or the reimbursement of services rendered by a publicly-run health centre through private health insurance.

However, this simple classification of the private/public mix can be misleading when more complex forms of ownership and corporate governance are considered. With stronger involvement of the private sector and the inflow of private capital there could be public facilities with partly private ownership. Conversely, private hospitals that are public contractors may receive funding from public sources and in turn have to comply with public sector regulations.

While private providers are playing a greater role in the delivery of services in many countries, there is clearly less scope for financing health services privately. Private health care markets fail to provide equitable health care and are inconsistent with many preventive and community-oriented goals. Governments must ensure that the overall public health goals and provision of health services to the poor are not endangered by cooperation with the private sector.

New public management and reforms of the health sector

Generally, government can take responsibility for organizing finance, service provision and regulation of health care organizations. Whether the state acts as provider or sees its role as the financer, or even solely as regulator, depends on the historical and political development of the health system. Where government health services occupy a large share of the market, the public health service is usually one of the largest public sector organizations in the country. However, the way in which public sector organizations operate has come under scrutiny and to many observers it appears that the public sector is less effective than the private in combating inefficiencies, such as waste of resources, low output and poor service quality (Mills *et al.* 2001).

These challenges have been addressed in the reforms the public sector has experienced in many countries over the last decades. Generally these reforms aim to improve government's capacity to mobilize revenue, set spending priorities and allocate and use resources effectively. Many of the ideas and approaches are related to financial management and have been adopted from the private sector. They have become known under the concept of *new public management* (NPM), which is founded on six principles (Hood 1995):

1 *Reorganizing the public sector into more autonomous, corporatized units.* Large organizations are decentralized and hospitals and local authorities are granted greater flexibility and autonomy in financial management. The overarching trend is to separate finance, service provision and regulation into separate and more autonomous organizational entities. Governments increasingly separate the functions of financing from providing health services (the purchaser-provider split) and also delegate powers to regulators and other public bodies with statutory responsibilities.
2 *Introduction of market elements with contract-based competitive provision.* Market elements are introduced within the overall structure of public services with the aim of increasing efficiency and consumer choice. These market arrangements are called internal or planned markets as they take place under the overall umbrella of the public organization. Purchasers of care may have a choice between a greater number of competing providers who offer services at lower prices or better quality. Patients may be offered the choice between different providers for treatment. Contract-based, performance-related reimbursements may replace traditional forms of resource allocation.
3 *Cooperation with the private sector and privatization.* The relationship between the public and private sector is characterized by a range of activities, such as private/public partnerships for capital investments, compulsory competitive tendering, partial (outsourcing) or complete privatization of public services. NGOs and private hospitals are becoming part of the provider network and operate on the same terms and contracts as public providers.

4 *Private-sector styles of management practice.* Private sector standards of accounting and financial reporting are now widely used in the public sector. Principles of corporate governance have been adopted from the private sector. Efforts are made to avoid waste of resources and to manage organizations effectively with emphasis on responsiveness to consumers. These changes entail a shift in corporate culture and leadership style from bureaucratic hierarchies to team orientation.

5 *Explicit use of measurable standards and measures of performance.* Financial reporting standards, methods of controlling and monitoring have been adopted from the private sector. At the organizational level, comparison of performance with regional and national data is increasingly used. At the political level, effective stewardship is seen as a key function of government, which involves devising overall strategies, setting quality standards and enforcing regulations. A key task of stewardship is assessing and monitoring the performance of the health system and using the evidence to communicate with stakeholders and as a basis for policy decisions.

6 *Greater emphasis on outcomes.* Accountability of clinicians and managers for outcomes plays an increasing role. Outcome data of the organization can be compared with regional or national data and used for decision-making. Methods of audit and quality management ensure that agreed targets are achieved.

Regulating financial autonomy

So far you have considered the roles of government as purchaser and as provider of health care. However, one of its central roles is regulating health services. This means setting and enforcing the rules under which health care organizations operate. Regulation may concern a range of issues such as access to care, quality, prices, capacity, service mix, levels of staffing and opening hours.

The financial incentives given to providers will largely depend on the regulations concerning the *residual claimant status* – that is, the use of the surplus or losses achieved in balancing income with expenditure. In economic theory, the term 'residual claimant' refers to who can retain the remaining surplus (or has to bear the financial loss) after all financial obligations of the firm, such as to pay staff, suppliers, bank interest and taxes, have been met. For example, in regulating the residual claimant status, government may set rules determining to what extent a hospital is permitted to keep any surplus or is held responsible for a loss.

The regulations for private sector organizations are often linked to tax status. The surplus is taxed if taken as a profit, or exempted from tax if reinvested in the corporation. If the company makes a loss, tax relief may be granted. Public sector organizations may be permitted to use the surplus for reinvesting in the organization. In contrast, if the surplus is retained by central government, provider managers have less incentive to use funds efficiently. Where the health system is based on contracts with both public and private sector providers, equal incentives should be given to both. Internationally, there are large differences as to the financial autonomy of providers and the extent to which private sector organizations are considered as equal partners in delivering care.

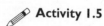 **Activity 1.5**

> What is the residual claimant status of your organization?

 Feedback

> There is a range of possible financial arrangements concerning the use of the surplus of an organization. While private sector organizations keep the amount of income that exceeds expenditure as a profit from which tax is deducted, not for profit organizations are usually exempted from tax, if they reinvest any surplus. Public sector organizations vary widely in the degree of financial autonomy and residual claimant status. Either the surplus is retained by government or they may have the discretion to reinvest the surplus fully or in part or to keep it as a reserve for future losses.

Summary

Financial management aims to ensure that health care resources are used in an appropriate way. You examined the basic input, process and outcome model and the economic, political, social and legal environment in which health care organizations operate. The main influencing factors considered in this chapter are the mechanisms of financing health care, the methods of provider payment and the institutional context under the public/private mix. You also examined the type of financial autonomy granted to provider organizations and how this affects management decisions. Finally, you looked at the principles shaping the reform of public services and the role that new approaches to financial management have played in managing public health care organizations.

References

Barnum, H., Kutzin, J. and Saxenian, H. (1995) *Incentives and Provider Payment Methods*, HRO Working Paper No. 51. Washington, DC: World Bank.

Briggs, C.J., Capdegelle, P. and Garner, P. (2002) Strategies for integrating primary health services in middle- and low-income countries: effects on performance, costs and patient outcomes (Cochrane Review), in *The Cochrane Library*, Issue 2. Oxford: Update Software.

Cassels, A. (1997) Aid instruments and health systems development: an analysis of current practice, *Health Policy and Planning*, 11(4): 254–68.

Donaldson, C. and Gerard, K. (1993) *Economics of Health Care Financing: The Visible Hand*. London: Macmillan.

Hood, C. (1995) The 'New Public Management' in the 1980s: variations on a theme, *Accounting, Organisations and Society*, 20(213): 93–109.

Mbandwa, L., Loewenson, R., Ropi, F., Sikosana, P., Zigora, T. and Chikumbirike, T. (2001) *Stakeholder Views on Resource Allocations in Health*, document commissioned by Zimbabwe Equity Gauge Project, MoHCW and TARSC. TARSC MoHCW EQUITY GAUGE Monograph 1/2001. Harare: July 2001.

McPake, B., Kumaranayake, L. and Normand, C. (2002) *Health Economics: An International Perspective*. London: Routledge.

Mills, A., Bennett, S. and Russell, S. (2001) Health sector reform and the role of government, in *The Challenge of Health Sector Reform: What Must Governments Do?* Basingstoke: Palgrave.

WHO (World Health Organization) (1995) *Changes in Sources of Finance*, Technical Report Series 829. Geneva: WHO.

2 | Financial and management accounting

Overview

In this chapter you will be introduced to the different roles of the finance department and explore in more detail what it means to make the best possible use of resources. You will look at the differences between financial and management accounting and examine the key elements of the annual budget cycle.

Learning objectives

By the end of this chapter you should be able to:

- **distinguish between the concepts of economy, efficiency and effectiveness**
- **examine how financial and management accounting contribute to financial management**
- **outline the annual budget cycle**
- **explain why financial management is important for your job**

Key terms

Balance sheet A statement of the total assets, liabilities and capital of an organization at a given moment.

Budget cycle The annual sequence of planning, budgeting, controlling and reporting to enable decisions on how an organization will use its resources.

Cash flow statement A statement summarizing the inflows and outflows of cash over the accounting period.

Economy Purchasing resources at least cost.

Effectiveness The extent to which an intervention produces a beneficial result under usual conditions of clinical care.

Financial accounting Financial information for external users reflecting the performance and financial standing of the organization.

Income statement (income and expenditure account) A summary of income and expenditure over the accounting period.

Operational (technical, productive) efficiency Using only the minimum necessary resources to finance, purchase and deliver a particular activity or set of activites (ie avoiding waste)

Management accounting Information for internal users to help them run the organization such as budgets, plans, costings and financial appraisals of service developments.

Treasury management Activities ensuring the organization has enough cash to meet all its financial obligations.

Making best use of resources

As you have seen in Chapter 1, financial management is concerned with questions that are important for any organization seeking to make the best use of its resources. But what is meant by 'best use of resources'? There are three principles – economy, effectiveness and efficiency – which are implicitly part of the appropriateness of any financial decision.

*   *Economy* is related to input and means doing things at least cost. Take for example the construction of a new health centre. As a manager, you will ask yourself whether it will cost more than is necessary. Obviously this is only meaningful when a basis of comparison is used. So you would compare the cost of the building to a facility of similar size or to planned costs. Similarly you would buy inputs such as drugs and medical supplies from the cheapest available source, if quality is equal.
*   *Effectiveness* is related to outcome. It means that the desired or expected outcome was achieved or, in other words, that the right thing was done. A newly-constructed health centre could still be effective, even if the building costs were higher than anticipated. But if for lack of funds an essential unit, such as the laboratory, was not built, the facility might be less effective than planned (or it may even be useless). Similarly, medical interventions must provide the expected benefit in order to be effective. Once again effectiveness is a relative measure which allows comparison of more and less effective ways of doing things.
*   *Efficiency* is an integrated measure of input process and outcome, and means doing things right. It can be measured by the ratio of process to input – for example, the number of patients treated per doctor – or quite often as input and outcome – for example, the cost per unit of outcome. You can compare efficiency over time or between organizations: for example, health centre A is more efficient than health centre B, or health centre C has improved efficiency during the last year; treatment X for cancer is more efficient than treatment Y. Generally, efficiency can be improved by increasing process or outcome for the same level of input or by decreasing input for the same level of process or outcome. Since efficiency is a ratio, you may also consider the proportionate changes of the two components: efficiency increases if the proportionate increase of outcome is greater than the proportionate increase of input and, vice versa, if the proportionate decrease of input is greater than the proportionate decrease of outcome (Jones and Pendlebury 1992).

✎ Activity 2.1

Write down some examples of how the concepts of economy, effectiveness and efficiency apply in your organization.

Activity 2.2

Suppose a Ministry of Health has received three bids on a tender for vaccinating children in a district.

Provider 1
Input: $3000
Process: 6000 vaccinations

Provider 2
Input: $4000
Process: 8800 vaccinations

Provider 3
Input: $6000
Process: 9000 vaccinations

How would you compare the efficiency of the three bids?

 Feedback

	Provider 1	Provider 2	Provider 3
Input ($)	3000	4000	6000
Process (no. of vaccinations)	6000	8800	9000
Input/process ($/vaccination)	0.5	0.45	0.67

This is straightforward and you would choose the provider who offers the lowest costs per unit of process. In real terms these choices can be difficult, because you need to have complete information about the alternative offers. The problem with this kind of comparison is that usually information on quality and similarity of standards needs to be defined thoroughly to be able to compare like with like.

Economy can apply to the purchase of consumables. However, if applied too far, cheap inputs may have an impact on service quality. The conflict arises where purchasing objectives to buy as cheaply as possible are reported separately from the services that are supplied where the outcomes may be adversely affected.

Effectiveness is normally measured by achieved outcomes or by comparing achieved outcomes to a desired level of effectiveness (e.g. reduction in tooth decay caused by a dental health education campaign or comparing breast cancer survival rates of your hospital to rates of all hospitals of the region).

Another way of describing efficiency is *value for money* (VFM), a term which is frequently used in financial management of public services. You would expect that a health care organization obtains VFM, or operates efficiently, if it attains its objectives at least cost and thus produces a maximum level of activity of the desired quality at a minimum level of waste or expense.

Efficiency measures will vary from organization to organization. There is nothing inherently wrong with this but, taken at its worst, it implies a narrow and rigid pursuit of existing performance standards without considering whether these are really worth achieving or could be improved. You as a manager will need to understand and apply all these concepts and make decisions on how to compromise if there is conflict between them. All these approaches are relevant to managing performance and each has an appropriate role to play in different situations.

The work of the finance department

Although this book is not intended to equip you with the skills necessary to become an accountant, you should, by the end of it, have a sound understanding of the types of information produced by your finance department and the purposes for which this information is used. In this chapter the three most important roles of the finance department – financial accounting, management accounting and cash management – are briefly introduced.

- *Financial accounting* provides summary accounts for external users and for regulatory bodies. It involves the recording of all monetary transactions and the production of summary financial statements that reflect the performance and financial standing of the organization. You will be returning to the area of financial accounting and the financial statements in Chapters 9 to 14.
- *Management accounts* provide financial information internally for managers to help them run the organization. This includes budgets and plans, costings and financial appraisal of service developments. Activities relating to management accounting are discussed in Chapters 3 to 8 and 15 to 20.
- *Cash management* involves ensuring the organization has enough cash to meet all of its current obligations. Money that is currently not used should not be left 'lying idle' in accounts on which no interest is paid. It also involves raising loans or some other form of finance to meet the organization's need for cash, when sufficient funds are not available, and planning long-term capital requirements – for example, for new facilities and equipment – and deciding on capital investments and how they should be financed. This cash management function is commonly referred to as *treasury management*. To perform this role effectively, the finance department will need detailed information from departmental managers on their planned levels of activity and the level and timing of cash flows both into and out of the organization, which are likely to result from the planned activity. You will find some more information on cash management in Chapter 13.

Other roles of the finance department include risk management, credit control, purchase ledger, payroll and compliance (ensuring that all financial regulations are met). Risk management entails activities related to risks that arise from entrepreneurial and clinical activities. Internal controls are used to analyse risk and avoid any financial overexposure. Insurance is usually taken out to cover against clinical negligence. Specific risks may arise from adverse exchange rates for foreign currency and inflation. Other activities of the finance department aim to improve performance in related areas of management such as logistics, supply chain management, buildings and establishment, market testing and contract management for outsourcing of service areas such as cleaning, catering, security and information technology.

Financial and management accounting

Table 2.1 shows some of the differences between financial and management accounting. You should note, though, that the information from financial accounts that summarize past performance is also used in setting plans and budgets, which are effectively an internal breakdown of the summary accounts. In addition, financial accounts can be analysed to give valuable insights into the comparative performance of similar organizations or of the same organization in different years. The two main statements of financial accounts are: the *balance sheet*, which reflects what the organization was worth (what it owned, what was owing to it, and what it owed to others) on a particular date, and the *income statement*, which summarizes the revenue and expenditure of the organization over the accounting period. A third statement, the *cash flow statement*, reflects the cash flows into and out of the organization over the accounting period, thus reconciling the cash position at the beginning of the accounting period with that at the end. You will learn about these statements in Chapters 9 to 14.

Table 2.1 The differences between financial and management accounting

Type of information	Management accounting Internal	Financial accounting External
Users	Managers	Supervisory board, government, stakeholders, shareholders
Purpose	Planning, monitoring, controlling	Score-keeping, giving a true and fair view of the organization
Time period	Monthly, quarterly, six-monthly, several years as appropriate	One year
Reports/statements	Budgets, activity forecasts, cost and investment appraisals	Income and expenditure, balance sheet, cash flow statement
Governed by	Needs of the organization	Legal requirements

Source: adapted from Allen and Myddleton (1992)

Management accounting

Management accounting is an important basis of decision-making. It provides the tools for evaluating, analysing, interpreting and judging the performance of the organization. It combines financial information with information on inputs and process, thus combining financial aspects with activity levels.

According to Pettinger (1994), the key purposes of management accounting relate to assessment and monitoring of:

- *Costs:* this relates to the question of how much it costs to produce the service and whether the level of resources used is appropriate. Managers will analyse costs by different categories and the improvements in economy that can be made.
- *Income:* managers are concerned with the sustainable inflow of funds to keep the organization going, and the mobilization of new sources of income.
- *Returns:* managers will seek to achieve a satisfactory surplus in relation to costs, activity or investment. Income needs to be balanced with costs, in such a way that returns are adequate to the type of organization and to its goals and comply with planned levels of activity.

Depending on the objectives of the organization, there may be more areas in which management accounting is required, for example, in managing projects, comparing performance or analysing market shares. You should note that management accounts are not confined to a one-year period in the same way as financial accounts. You may consider shorter or longer periods of time than one year, as appropriate. For example, weekly, monthly or quarterly reports are used in monitoring costs and activity, longer periods of time are used for business plans, government five-year plans and the long-term analysis of returns on investment.

The budget cycle

Budgets provide information on future expenditure which will assist managers in planning, monitoring and controlling operations. In large organizations central budgets can be devolved to unit managers who are responsible for the resources entrusted to them. The extent of devolution may vary: central government funds may be devolved to regions and from there to providers in districts, and within larger institutions, such as hospitals, to departments and units. Accountability is established through giving managers responsibility for achieving performance targets based on the information provided by the budget.

Planning, budgeting, controlling and reporting are the key elements of the annual budget cycle (see Figure 2.1), in which the decisions are made as to how the organization will use its resources (Jones and Pendlebury 1992). *Planning* is concerned with forecasting both future activity and resource levels. *Activity planning* makes decisions about the expected level of activity – for example, numbers of vaccinations to be performed or cases to be treated. *Resource planning* arranges for adequate inputs for the planned activity – for example, the funds required to pay staff and equipment to achieve the set service goals. A useful distinction can be made between *strategic planning* and *operational planning*. Strategic planning is concerned with the long-term, overall aims and objectives of the organization. Operational planning puts long-term objectives into practice. The overall aims and objectives are broken down into a series of manageable objectives and a set of activities to be performed within a time frame of up to one year.

In the *budget stage* all inputs identified as necessary by operational planning for the coming year are expressed in monetary terms. Thus the budget lists the monetary

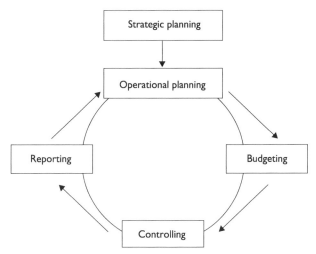

Figure 2.1 The budget cycle

values of the inputs in such a way that all staff in charge can easily understand the types and values of the resources used in the organization. The budget is the blueprint for managing expenditure according to set categories such as staff, supplies, equipment, energy and so on. Once the budget is approved, the budget-holder is permitted to spend the money according to set limits and rules.

Controlling and monitoring ensures that activity and use of resources stay within planned limits. Actual activity and spending are monitored continuously and compared to budgeted activity and spending levels. Achieving planned levels of income and expenditure at the end of the year is not the only objective. Spending on line items (such as staff, drugs and supplies) must comply with the appropriate combination of inputs. Both over- and underspending on single items such as staff, drugs or supplies can affect the performance of the organization without changing the overall balance. However, total overspending has severe consequences for running the organization and may lead to closing operations if the deficit cannot be compensated.

Reporting refers to variance analysis and feedback: reasons for the variance (difference) between actual and scheduled spending need to be identified and reported to the responsible level of management. As there are many causes for a deviation of actual from planned figures, a careful analysis has to be performed. The reports need to be timely and accurate in order to enable managers to take corrective actions. Possible reasons for variance can be internal or external to the organization. For example, changes in demand or increases in the price of supplies are external; mismanagement and waste of resources are internal causes. Management must take the appropriate corrective action such as adjusting activity or spending levels and adjusting the operational objectives for the following year.

Why financial management is important in your job

So far you have seen why financial management is important to running health care organizations and that sound financial skills are required in assessing costs and monitoring budgets. You may also think of other challenges for the finance department such as deciding on a new technology or identifying the impact of opening a new department, appraising the returns on an investment or the consequences of closing a health centre.

 Activity 2.3

Why is financial management important for you in your job?

1 Identify at least three occasions in recent weeks when you have needed to make financial management decisions.
2 Think of your organization and list those questions that management accounting can help resolve. (Your list should refer to actual issues faced by the organization – it should not be a generic list.)

 Feedback

1 The decisions you identified will be unique to you. While in health care the focus is on the patient, all decisions made within a health service involve resource use and therefore have financial management implications.

2 The scope of the questions you identify should be as broad as possible covering both your unit and the whole organization. They are likely to include questions on the:

• cost of services in your organization
• cost of activities in your organization
• cost of patient treatments
• cost of developing services
• replacement of equipment

If you cannot identify a substantial list then it is worth talking to your colleagues to identify what the main concerns are. If you know these then you are really in touch with what is going on in your organization.

Summary

Financial management is an essential management skill that enables managers to make the best use of resources. Financial accounting provides summary accounts in prescribed formats for external users of accounts and for regulatory bodies. The two main statements of account are:

• the balance sheet, which reflects what the organization was worth (i.e. what it owns, what is owing to it and what it owes to others) on a particular date;

- the income statement, which summarizes the revenue and expenditure of the organization over the accounting period.

A third statement, the cash flow statement, reflects the cash flows into and out of the business over the accounting period, thus reconciling the cash position at the beginning of the accounting period with that at the end.

Management accounting is intended for internal purposes; its objective is to provide managers with information for decision-making and control purposes. Costing information is used by managers to make informed pricing decisions and to set budgets which are the basis for management planning and control. In the following chapters you will move on to learn about costing.

References

Allen, M.W. and Myddleton, D.R. (1992) *Essential Management Accounting*. London: Prentice Hall Europe.

Jones, R. and Pendlebury, M. (1992) *Public Sector Accounting*. London: Pitman.

Pettinger, R. (1994) *Introduction to Management*. London: Macmillan.

SECTION 2

Management accounting

3 | The nature of costs

Overview

If there is one key financial skill you need as a manager it is an awareness of costs and how these vary with activity. This chapter examines the different types of costs and how they vary, and applies this in a health care setting to patient costs.

You will first see how to define costs and look at different uses of cost information before considering the behaviour of different cost categories and applying them to preparing a flexible budget and constructing cost profiles for defined groups of patients.

Learning objectives

By the end of this chapter you should be able to:

- **describe how different costs behave**
- **explain and project how costs vary with level of activity**
- **apply cost information to prepare a flexible budget and cost profiles**

Key terms

Cost profile A typical pattern of the costs associated with a category of patient or group of patients.

Financial (budgetary) cost The accounting cost of a good or service usually representing the original (historical) amount paid, distinct from the opportunity cost.

Fixed cost A cost of production that does not vary with the level of output.

Flexible budget A budget showing comparative costs for a range of levels of activity.

Opportunity (economic) cost The value of the next best alternative forgone as a result of the decision made.

Semi-variable costs Costs that contain both a fixed and a variable element.

Stepped costs Costs that behave like fixed costs until certain thresholds are reached; when activity increases beyond each threshold, costs step to a higher level and remain fixed until the next threshold level of activity is reached.

Variable costs A cost of production that varies directly with the level of output.

Some important distinctions

Before embarking on a discussion of costs it is worth making some important distinctions. When financial managers refer to costs they are referring to:

• *Financial cost:* the monetary value of resources (inputs).

This should not be confused with:

• *Opportunity (economic) cost:* the full cost (of an illness, an intervention etc.) borne by society, based on opportunity cost (the income or benefit foregone as a result of carrying out a particular decision), regardless of whether the resources were purchased or not.

In this book you will be concerned only with financial costs. It is also important to be clear that there is often a difference between cost in monetary terms and the value that is placed on costs. Sometimes it is difficult to put a monetary value on a cost – for example, when you are considering intangible cost such as pain and suffering. Financial costs aim only to measure *monetary values*.

You should also note that it is important that you do not mix up the terms *costs* and *resources*:

• *resources* are the inputs required for a production process;
• *costs* measure the *value* of the resources.

Defining costs

Financial managers can present cost information in many different ways and a different definition of cost is needed to cover each of these aspects. Take for example the cost of a car that is used in a vaccination campaign. You could look at its replacement cost, the price the programme manager paid three years ago, the cost of leasing instead of buying a new car, or you could assess how the car affects fixed, variable and marginal campaign costs. (You will be learning about fixed, variable and marginal costs in this chapter.)

What is a cost and why are there so many different ways of measurement? Costs can be defined as the value of the resources used in the production of an item or service. From this you can see that it is not only the money that changes hands when an item is bought that is regarded as a cost: a number of different types of cost and ways of measuring costs can be identified. These include:

• *historical cost,* which is the amount of money paid for the resources used;
• *replacement cost,* which is what it would cost in today's money to replace the resources that have been used;
• *full cost,* which includes both the costs directly associated with the production of the service and costs that would be incurred whether or not the activity was carried out;
• *marginal cost,* which is the additional cost of producing one additional unit of a service;
• *purchase cost,* which is what it would cost to pay an external organization to produce the service on your behalf (e.g. what it would cost to use an external laboratory to carry out blood tests).

You can see that none of these types of cost is 'better' than any of the others. The answer to which is the most appropriate will depend on the purposes for which the cost information is required.

 Activity 3.1

Reflect on what is meant by each part of the definition: 'Costs are the value of the resources used in the production of a service'.

 Feedback

This definition suggests that costs are not just cash flow. A monetary loss may not only occur when a resource is acquired but also while it is consumed. Some resources are used up quickly and frequently such as stocks and consumables and staff time or labour. Other resources, such as buildings and equipment, are used slowly and over a longer period of time.

Reasons for measuring costs

There are three main reasons for which accountants measure costs:

1 *for stock and asset valuation* for financial accounting purposes (you will learn more about this in Chapters 9 to 11;
2 *for decision-making purposes*, enabling managers to reach informed decisions as to whether to offer a service, what prices to charge, etc.
3 *for control purposes* so that budgets can be constructed and activity can be monitored against budgets.

In each case a different range of cost classifications is used. This chapter focuses on accounting for decision-making and control.

In health services the following are typical of decisions where there is a need for accurate, relevant and timely information, which is interpreted correctly:

• Should we appoint a new consultant anaesthetist?
• Should we close this ward?
• Should we run outpatient clinics from a different location?
• Should we contract an outside supplier to provide cleaning services?

In health services there will also be other considerations than cost to be taken into account: public health and environmental implications of a decision and the clinical freedom of doctors are examples. However, a knowledge of the associated costs will remain essential for an appreciation of the consequences of alternative courses of action.

Activity 3.2

Spend a few minutes thinking about and making notes on the cost information that is used by a health service or an area within a heath service with which you are familiar. For what purposes is this cost information used?

Feedback

The cost information you have listed will probably be wide-ranging and may include staff costs, equipment costs, the costs of disposable supplies, cleaning costs, maintenance and repairs, administration costs and many others.

In health services the main uses of reliable and accurate cost information include:

- *resource allocation:* in developing a budget it is necessary to know the cost of its components; if you understand the costs of services, such as hospitals and health centres, you can develop budgets and allocate resources to each area of activity within the service
- *comparison:* you can compare costs between hospitals, health centres, districts or regions and develop performance indicators such as cost per capita, cost per hospital bed
- *evaluation:* cost information is essential when you want to determine the best value for money
- *monitoring and control:* at institutional level, cost information is the basis of assessing financial performance
- *pricing:* cost information is the basis of pricing; providers of health services need to know the cost of services they supply and purchasers need accurate information on the cost of the services they are going to demand

How do costs behave?

Consider now the relationship between cost and activity. As a manager, in order to stand some chance of managing your budget, you need an awareness of costs and how these vary with activity. In addition, if you know your costs for various activities, then you are in a position to take decisions on who should provide services. For instance, is it cheaper to do something in-house or should the activity be subcontracted?

Health services require many different types of resources such as buildings, equipment, staff time and drugs. The costs of a specific service depend on:

- the resources employed (the resource mix);
- the quantity of each resource required.

By definition all resources incur a cost when they are employed. If the level of activity stays constant, costs won't change. If the level of activity increases, costs will change but the extent to which this happens is not straightforward. Resources have different characteristics in the way they affect cost when activity changes. The way in which costs respond to changes in activity is called *cost behaviour.*

How much a service costs at different levels of activity depends on the cost behaviour of its inputs. Managers normally group the resources into categories according to how their consumption changes with activity. These categories are:

- variable;
- fixed;
- semi-variable;
- stepped.

Variable costs

Variable costs are those which change simultaneously with activity. When activity increases, costs go up; when activity decreases, costs go down. Examples include the costs of meals prepared, which will change in direct proportion to the number of beds occupied and the number of drugs issued which, under a relatively stable case mix, will vary in proportion to the number of patients treated.

Table 3.1 shows the cost of drugs in an outpatient clinic as an example of variable costs, and Figure 3.1 is a graphical illustration of how variable costs behave.

Table 3.1 Variable costs

Number of patients treated	2 180	2 433
Cost of drugs	$109 000	$121 650
Average cost of drugs per patient/unit of activity	$50	$50

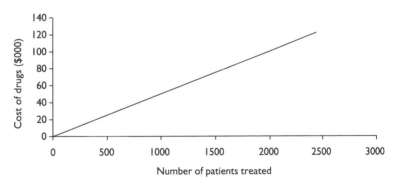

Figure 3.1 Variable cost graph

Fixed costs

Fixed costs are those which stay constant with changes in activity over a period of time. The costs of resources which must be paid for before any activity occurs but which stay fixed as activity increases are fixed costs. Examples include staff salaries (of permanent staff) and buildings' maintenance.

Table 3.2 shows some of the fixed costs for the outpatient clinic mentioned above.

Note that these costs will be incurred whether or not the clinic treats a single patient.

Table 3.2 Fixed costs

Rent	$10 000
Equipment maintenance and repairs	$3 000
Administration costs	$15 000
Total fixed costs	$28 000

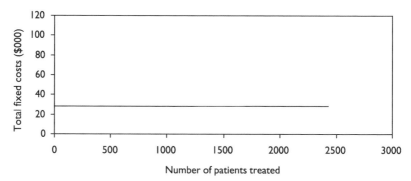

Figure 3.2 Fixed costs graph

The fixed cost per unit of activity in this example is calculated by dividing the total fixed costs by the number of patients treated. Thus:

- if 2180 patients were treated, the average fixed cost per patient would be: 28,000 ÷ 2180 = $12.84;
- if 2433 patients were treated, the average fixed cost per patient would be: 28,000 ÷ 2433 = $11.51.

Note that in the long run all costs will vary – the rental can be cancelled on premises no longer required or larger premises may be acquired, equipment no longer in use may be sold off or new equipment may be bought, and so on. The shorter the period of time the greater the number of costs that are likely to be fixed.

Semi-variable costs

Some costs contain both a fixed and a variable element; these are known as semi-variable costs. These arise where resources incur a standing charge that is payable regardless of whether the input is used plus a variable cost when activity increases. Utility bills such as those for telephone and electricity are examples: they include both a fixed rental charge and a charge determined by the level of usage of the utility.

Table 3.3 Semi-variable costs

Number of patients treated	2 180	2 433
Semi-variable costs	($00)	($00)
Telephone charges	$2 850	$3 100
Electricity	$3 300	$3 500
Photocopying	$500	$600
Total semi-variable costs	$6 650	$7 200
Average cost per patient	$3.05	$2.96

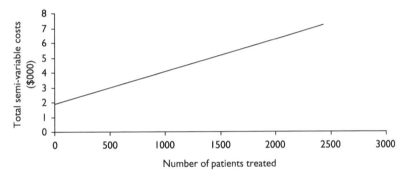

Figure 3.3 Semi-variable cost graph

Stepped costs

Stepped costs behave like fixed costs but only until a certain threshold is reached. When activity increases further, costs step to a higher level. This process continues as activity increases. In the example of the outpatient clinic, certain costs will be fixed regardless of the level of activity, whereas others may increase significantly once a certain level of activity is reached. Once certain levels of activity are reached it will, for example, be necessary to employ another member of staff and the associated costs will 'step up' to a new level. Other examples of resources with stepped costs are rentals, equipment and machinery.

In the example of the outpatient clinic that you have been following, it may be necessary to take on an additional nurse when the number of patients treated reaches 2400. The salary for the additional staff member is $10,000. The effect of this is shown in Figure 3.4 and Table 3.4 shows the effect of this step in costs on the cost per patient.

Table 3.4 Staff costs

Number of patients treated	2 180	2 399	2 400	2 433
Staff costs	$60 000	$60 000	$70 000	$70 000
Average staff costs per patient	$27.52	$25.01	$29.16	$28.77

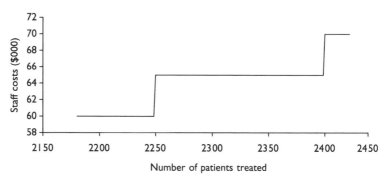

Figure 3.4 Stepped costs graph

Activity 3.3

To check your understanding of the different cost behaviours, categorize the following resources of a health centre into fixed, variable, semi-variable and stepped costs: drugs, doctors, telephone, X-ray equipment, laboratory assistant, appliances, general manager, building, nurses, X-ray plates.

Feedback

1 Fixed costs: X-ray equipment, general manager, building.

2 Variable costs: drugs, appliances, X-ray plates.

3 Semi-variable costs: telephone.

4 Stepped costs: doctors, nurses, laboratory assistant.

Total cost

Total cost is the total of fixed, variable, semi-variable and stepped costs for a particular level of activity. Once you have identified and analysed all of the different costs you can work out total costs at a given level of activity.

Activity 3.4

Assume that Tables 3.1, 3.2, 3.3 and 3.4 above show all of the variable, fixed, semi-variable and stepped costs for the clinic and that no other costs are incurred.

Calculate the total costs for the clinic described above when:

1 2180 patients are treated
2 2433 patients are treated.

Feedback

The costs for treatment of 2180 and 2433 patients respectively are as shown in Table 3.5.

Table 3.5 Total cost calculation

Number of patients treated	2 180	2 433
	$	$
Variable costs	109 000	121 650
Fixed costs	28 000	28 000
Semi-variable costs	6 650	7 200
Stepped costs	60 000	70 000
Total costs	203 650	226 850

Using cost information for flexible budgets

Given the total costs at a given level of activity, you can calculate the average unit cost. In the example of the outpatient clinic, the cost per patient at each of the given levels of activity is:

- 203,650 ÷ 2180 = $93.42
- 226,850 ÷ 2433 = $93.24

This approach is useful in preparing a *flexible budget*, a budget showing comparative costs for a range of levels of activity, as you will see in the following activity.

Activity 3.5

An environmental health laboratory is performing 1000 analyses of air pollution per year. Its income varies with the number of tests performed and was $60,000 in the last year. The Ministry of Health wants to increase the number of analyses from next year. The equipment is fairly new and runs below its capacity, but sample processing is labour intensive and one laboratory assistant can handle only up to 1000 analyses per year. The average salary of a laboratory assistant is $15,000 per year. You are asked to set up a flexible budget for 2000, 3000 and 4000 tests per annum, based on the information set out in Table 3.6. For the purposes of this activity you should assume that income increases in a straight line (in direct proportion to activity).

Table 3.6 Budget cost sheet for 2000, 3000 and 4000 tests per annum

Number of tests	Fixed costs ($)	Stepped costs ($)	Variable costs ($)	Total costs ($)	Total income ($)	Surplus (deficit) ($)
1 000	100 000	15 000	1 300		60 000	
2 000						
3 000						
4 000						

Feedback

You should have arrived at the figures shown in Table 3.7. (Brackets indicate a deficit.)

Table 3.7 Completed budget for 2000, 3000 and 4000 tests per annum

Number of tests	Fixed costs ($)	Stepped costs ($)	Variable costs ($)	Total costs ($)	Total income ($)	Surplus (deficit) ($)
1 000	100 000	15 000	1 300	116 300	60 000	(56 300)
2 000	100 000	30 000	2 600	132 600	120 000	(12 600)
3 000	100 000	45 000	3 900	148 900	180 000	31 100
4 000	100 000	60 000	5 200	165 200	240 000	74 800

A budget such as this that identifies the income and cost for the potential different levels of activity is known as a flexible budget. You will be returning to flexible budgeting in Chapters 7 and 8.

At current activity levels (1000 tests) the laboratory is already incurring a serious deficit; therefore there is a significant risk of underperformance, which will produce a financial deficit. At higher levels of activity a surplus is generated. However, the assumption that income increases in a straight line is probably unrealistic – in the real world it is more likely that deals will be negotiated and activity priced at marginal rates.

This example has shown the importance of fixed costs in management decisions. So if you have a fixed cost problem, if possible you should consider whether there is any way of cutting these (which can be a tough job) or of increasing activity levels to cover the fixed costs that you are stuck with in the short and medium term.

Average and marginal costs

You have already come across the concepts of average and marginal costs in this chapter. Average cost is calculated by dividing total cost by the level or quantity of activity:

TC/Q

Activity 3.6

Work out, to the nearest $, the average cost for 1000, 2000, 3000, 4000 tests in the example above (Activity 3.5).

Feedback

Your answers should have been:

$116, $66, $50, $41

As you see, average costs are initially high because fixed costs are spread over a low level of activity; as activity rises then fixed costs are spread over more and more tests, reducing the average costs.

Marginal costs are the cost of producing one more unit of activity, for example the extra cost of moving from four tests to five. This can be calculated by the following formula:

$$\Delta TC/\Delta Q$$

where (ΔTC is the increase in total costs as a result of the fifth test and ΔQ is the increase in activity (in this case the additional test).

Marginal costs are useful in incremental analysis. For example, what are the costs of treating one more patient? In a simple example with just fixed cost and variable cost, marginal cost is equivalent to the increase in variable cost as activity rises.

Cost profiles

A different way of looking at costs is assessing *cost profiles* over time – for example, costs incurred by a patient with pneumonia during each day of a hospital stay or costs of a group of diabetes patients during each month of a year. Although every patient is unique, with different needs and different treatments, by careful groupings of patients by specialties and diagnoses it is possible to identify patients with similar treatment needs and estimate average costs for these groups. It will never be possible, or worthwhile, to cost every patient grouping; however, it is certainly possible to cost the more frequently-occurring and important conditions that contribute significantly to costs. This approach is also the basis of identifying DRGs.

The following summary, based on an example in Mellett *et al.* (1993), illustrates the use of cost profiles. Read through it carefully and make sure you follow the logic behind the calculations.

 Inpatient cost profiles

In a fully staffed and resourced general surgery ward with 40 beds the costs associated with each patient follow a typical pattern. On admission the patient is allocated a bed and during the first few days undergoes a number of tests and examinations followed by a surgical procedure or medical investigation after which they are prescribed a course of antibiotics. After this the patient may stay in hospital for a period of recovery, during which time they will be monitored and will receive assistance from nursing and other support staff. As time progresses they will need less support until they are discharged. Once the patient is discharged the bed remains empty for a period of time (known as the turnover interval) until a new patient is admitted; then the cost pattern will be repeated. The costs associated with this pattern are shown in Figure 3.5.

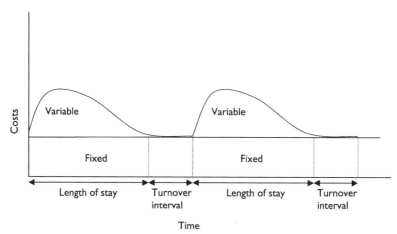

Figure 3.5 Cost profile for surgical ward inpatients

Source: Adapted from Mellett et al. (1993: 93)

From Figure 3.5 you can see that the total costs associated with each patient include both fixed costs which remain constant over time and variable costs which peak at the time of surgery then tail off to the time when the patient is discharged. The cost profile is the same for each patient, so the total cost of a series of patients is the total cost of a typical stay multiplied by the number of patients. However, this does not take account of the fixed costs that are incurred during the turnover interval when the hospital bed is empty.

Records show that in a 52-week period the total number of patients, treated was 2080 and that this group of patients remained in hospital for a total of 10,400 days.

The average length of stay (ALOS) can be calculated as:

Total hospital days ÷ number of patients treated

10,400 ÷ 2080 = 5 days

The turnover interval is obtained by dividing the total number of days for which beds remained vacant by the number of patients as follows:

Beds are available 52 weeks × 7 days × 40 beds = 14,560 days

Beds are occupied: 10,400 days

Therefore, days beds are unused   4,160

Turnover interval = unused bed days ÷ number of patients = 4160 ÷ 2080 = 2 days

The following cost information is also available:

Fixed costs $900,000

Variable costs $280,000

The cost per patient is calculated by taking the total costs (fixed costs plus variable costs) for the period and dividing this by the number of patients treated:

900,000 + 280,000 = 1,180,000 ÷ 2080 = $567 per patient

This cost per patient can also be calculated as follows:

Variable costs for the 52-week period	$280,000
Number of patients	2,080
Cost per patient (1)	$135
Fixed costs	$900,000
Number of bed days available	14,560
(Fixed) cost per day	$62
Cost per ALOS ($62 × 5) (2)	$309
Cost of two-day turnover interval (3)	$124
Total cost per patient = (1) + (2) + (3)	$568

(The difference of $1 in the cost per patient is due to rounding up to the nearest dollar in the calculations.)

From the second calculation it can be seen that the cost of the turnover interval is included in the cost per patient.

In the above example there are a number of measures that might be taken to reduce the cost per patient. The next activity asks you to work out how the cost per patient would be affected by reducing the turnover interval so that beds remain vacant for shorter periods, and by reducing the average length of stay per patient.

 Activity 3.7

1 Calculate the effect on the cost per patient of reducing the turnover interval from two days to one day in the above example, following these instructions:

   a) Calculate the number of patients who will be treated in a 52-week period if the turnover interval is reduced to one day
   b) Work out the total cost associated with the treatment of this increased number of patients
   c) Calculate the cost per patient.

2 Now assume that action is taken to reduce the average length of stay of this increased number of patients from five days to four. Calculate:

   a) the number of patients who will be treated in a 52-week period
   b) the total cost associated with the treatment of this increased number of patients
   c) the cost per patient.

Feedback

Your calculations should be as follows:

1 For a reduction in the turnover interval to one day:

a) Total available bed days = 14,560
 Average length of stay + turnover interval = 6 days
 Number of patients treated = 14,560 ÷ 6 = 2427
b) Total cost = fixed costs ($900,000) + variable costs (2427 × $135) = $900,000 +
 $327,645 = $1,227,645
c) Cost per patient = $1,227,645 ÷ 2427 = $506.

Note that the total cost of treating the increased number of patients increases since total variable costs increase with number of patients. However, because the fixed costs are being shared between more patients, the cost per patient is reduced.

2 If the average length of stay is then reduced from five to four days:

a) The number of patients treated will be total available bed days (14,560) divided by
 the average length of stay and turnover interval per patient (4 + 1 = 5 days) = 2912
 patients seen in a 52-week period
b) The total cost of treating 2912 patients will be fixed costs ($900,000) + variable
 costs (2912 × $135) = $900,000 + $393,120 = $1,293,120
c) Cost per patient = $1,293,120 ÷ 2912 = $444.

You can see from this exercise that increasing the turnover and reducing the average length of stay can have a dramatic effect on the cost per patient. However, you should be aware that changes in the turnover interval may often have a significant impact elsewhere in the system in terms of the organization's capacity to respond to peaks in emergency demand.

Cost profiles will vary according to the type of activity but the same principles as those illustrated in this summary can be applied in most areas of activity within health services.

Projecting costs

One of the most important challenges for managers is how to project or forecast the impact of changes in activity on financial performance. Managers need to prepare budgets based on estimated levels of activity and, when comparing actual results with the budget, they need to estimate again what the costs should have been for the actual levels of activity which were achieved. The problem is that the level of activity is difficult to predict because health care is highly complex and varies depending on patient needs, as you will see in the following chapters. For this reason, flexible budgets are prepared, using information about costs and their behaviour, to forecast for a range of activity levels. In Activity 3.5 you saw how flexible budgets are constructed; you will be returning to flexible budgets in Chapters 7 and 8.

Summary

Costs are the value of the resources used in the production of a service. How much a health service costs at different levels of activity depends on the cost behaviour of its resources. Dependent on how the consumption of a particular resource changes with activity, costs can be grouped into variable, fixed, semi-variable and stepped costs. Total cost is the sum of costs of all resources at a certain level of activity. This approach can be used in areas such as preparing a flexible budget and in constructing cost profiles. Preparing a flexible budget requires you to identify the income and expenditure for different levels of activity. Constructing cost profiles gives you an account of cost changes over time and allows you to assess total costs for defined patient groups with similar treatment needs to estimate average costs.

Reference

Mellett, H., Marriott, N. and Harries, S. (1993) *Financial Management in the NHS: A Manager's Handbook*. London: Chapman & Hall.

4

The costing process

Overview

Managers need to be able to operate in complex organizations. Large organizations, such as hospitals performing a range of sophisticated services, are divided into units which can be considered as cost centres. Some of these units are directly involved in patient care – these are front-line units; others are support units providing services to front-line units. In this chapter you will look at the different ways in which costs can be identified and recorded to capture the complexity of a service and how this information can be used in decision-making.

Learning objectives

By the end of this chapter you should be able to:

- **describe the different ways of grouping and classifying costs**
- **explain how costs can be either allocated or apportioned to different service units**
- **justify which approach to apportionment of shared costs should be used**

Key terms

Cost allocation Charging an entire cost to the cost centre that is directly responsible for incurring it.

Cost apportionment Sharing a central cost between cost centres in proportion to the level of use each cost centre makes of it.

Cost centre Any activity or unit of organization for which you want to identify costs.

Direct costs Resources used in the design, implementation, receipt and continuation of a health care intervention.

Indirect costs The value of resources expended by patients and their carers to enable individuals to receive an intervention.

Overhead costs Costs that are not incurred directly from providing patient care but are necessary to support the organization overall (eg personnel functions).

Cost recording

In Chapter 3 you saw how costs change with activity levels and learned to distinguish between fixed, variable, semi-variable and stepped fixed costs. In this chapter you will look at a different aspect of costs – the ways in which they are classified. There are a number of different ways of classifying or describing costs but, with some exceptions, you will see that many of these descriptions relate to where the cost is incurred or recognized in the process of service delivery.

Why record costs?

Detailed cost records need to be kept for two important purposes:

1 *For management accounting:* to assist internal management decisions in the day-to-day operation of a health care organization and the planning and controlling of activity, for example by comparing current spending levels with the budget or with spending in previous years, or deciding whether to merge two wards.
2 *For financial accounting:* to enable the organization to produce financial statements in a specific format to meet the legal requirements set by government or supervisory bodies and to provide people outside the organization with detailed and true information about its financial situation.

A hospital which is recording, say, costs and activity for quarterly management accounts normally also produces a separate financial accounting report at the end of the year (the annual account) for its board or for government.

What is cost accounting?

Cost accounting is the process of determining either the full or the incremental costs of providing services to patients and other customers. It is important to ensure that no costs are overlooked in the process. Costs which are vital to the operation of a health service, even though they do not provide direct patient or customer services, must also be taken into consideration in determining these costs. When considering costs you need to specify clearly what unit or activity within the organization you are looking at. In other words, you need to specify clearly the *cost centre*. A cost centre is any activity or unit of organization for which you want to identify costs. It could be a front-line service, a support service, a department or even the costs incurred by a single patient. If cost centres are not carefully defined, the costs reported could be misinterpreted and lead to wrong conclusions.

How are costs recorded?

Accounts should not only give aggregate figures but should also provide detailed information on the various uses of expenditure. A common way of analysing health systems expenditure is to disaggregate spending into line items (also called subjective or input costs), functional costs and specialty costs. This way of splitting up costs gives detailed answers to the following questions:

- On *what* has the money been spent? (e.g. equipment, drugs, energy, capital charges) – line items.
- *Where* has it been spent? (e.g. on wards, outpatient clinics, catering) – functional costs.
- In *which specialty* has it been spent? (e.g. surgery, general medicine, gynaecology) – specialty costs.

Thus a number of dimensions can be used to define a single cost item, allowing you to break down each cost item to a detailed level – for example, a nurse's salary in a general medicine ward, or a doctor's salary in the psychiatric day clinic.

Cost coding systems

For recording costs of small organizations a simple system that will allow recording of expenditure in basic categories such as staff, equipment, drugs and consumables may be sufficient. Such a system may be set up using a basic spreadsheet or may even be entered in books of account known as ledgers. However, in large organizations with dozens of different activities and thousands of financial transactions, computerized accounting programs provide assistance. Such systems employ codes to assist in identifying and recording costs in such a way that they can be analysed along different dimensions, such as the three dimensions identified above. Thus, the code assigned to the salary of a nurse working in the outpatient clinic of the ophthalmology department would have three separate identifiers:

- nurse;
- ophthalmology;
- outpatient clinic.

This allows managers to include that nurse's salary when reviewing staff costs, the costs of the ophthalmology department and the costs of the outpatient clinic. In large organizations such coding systems can allow for the complex analysis of a vast amount of data with thousands of different cost codes. There are a number of accounting software packages designed specifically for this purpose.

A financial coding system allows financial managers to define minimum requirements for cost recording across organizations. If uniformly implemented by organizations within health systems, the coding system can assist in comparing costs between organizations. Coding provides additional security and accuracy since it ensures that the correct uses of each financial transaction are identified. Provided all transactions have been recorded properly you obtain a comprehensive picture of costs that can be analysed and displayed in many different ways.

Direct costs, indirect costs and overheads

Costs may also be classified into direct costs, indirect costs and overheads. For an assessment of the *financial* costs of a service a distinction is made between:

- *direct costs:* these are the costs of resources used directly by the service, for example, doctors, nurses, drugs;
- *indirect costs:* these are the services provided by support units, such as radiology and catering; indirect costs are related to resources that are common to many clinical treatments and which are normally supplied centrally to many users;
- *overhead costs:* these are costs that are not incurred directly from providing patient care but are necessary to support the organization overall, such as central management, security, accounting and housekeeping.

 Activity 4.1

Suppose you are a manager of an accident and emergency (A&E) department. From the following list identify five items which represent direct, indirect and overhead costs: nurses, cotton wool, laboratory tests, drugs, endotracheal tubes, drainage bags, scalpels, cannulae, telephones, staff travel, administrator, photocopying, accountancy and clerical officer, secretary, medical officer, estate administration, lighting, catering staff, X-ray department, clinical director, gauze bandages, printing and stationery, heating, kitchen.

 Feedback

Examples are as follows.

1 Direct costs: nurses, cotton wool, gauze bandages, drainage bags, drugs.

2 Indirect costs: clinical director, X-ray department, photocopying, laboratory tests, printing and stationery.

3 Overheads: accountancy and clerical officer, estate administration, heating, lighting, catering staff.

Apportioning shared costs

Indirect costs and overheads are shared resources. So you need to identify what part of these resources is consumed by the cost centre you are looking at. You should be aware of the technical difference between cost allocation and cost apportionment. Both are key techniques in costing and they focus on the distinction between direct and indirect costs or overheads.

Direct costs can be *allocated* directly; shared costs such as indirect costs and overheads need to be *apportioned*. Apportioning shared resources requires some information on the distribution of resource use and costs across cost centres. Where the cost of physical resources is being apportioned this may be on the basis of floor space occupied, time spent or some other basis.

Activity 4.2

1 Look at costs that are shared by the A&E department with other units. The hospital has performed 14,000 X-ray examinations at a cost of $1,000,000. Identify the shared cost to be apportioned to each department on the basis of the number of requests.

Table 4.1 X-rays performed by radiology department

Department	Number of requests	Costs ($)
A&E	1 200	
General medicine	2 500	
Surgery	3 000	
Renal	1 000	
Paediatrics	1 300	
Other	5 000	
Total	14 000	1 000 000

2 Next, look at the overheads for estate management. The hospital spends a total of $600,000 for estate management of a floor area of 29,000 m². How much would you apportion to A&E? How much would you apportion to each of the other departments?

Table 4.2 Estate management costs

Estates	Floor area (m²)	Costs ($)
A&E	2 500	
General medicine	4 000	
Surgery	5 000	
Renal	3 000	
Paediatrics	4 500	
Other	10 000	
Total	29 000	600 000

 Feedback

As you see, you need to have a clear understanding of inputs and processes of the service you are looking at in order to identify shared costs.

1 The A&E department's share of costs for X-rays is $85,714. You should have first calculated the unit cost of X-rays by dividing $1,000,000 by 14,000 to arrive at a figure of $71.43 per X-ray. Then you should have multiplied the unit cost by the number of requests for each department to arrive at the indirect cost of X-rays for each department, arriving at costs as indicated in the third column of Table 4.3.

Table 4.3 Costs of X-rays performed by radiology department

Radiology	Number of requests	Costs ($)
A&E	1 200	85 714
General medicine	2 500	178 571
Surgery	3 000	214 286
Renal	1 000	71 429
Paediatrics	1 300	92 857
Other	5 000	357 143
Total	14 000	1 000 000

2 The A&E department's shared cost of estate management is $51,724. In this case you needed to apportion costs according to the proportion of total floor space occupied. Thus you should have divided total estate management costs ($600,000) by total floor space (29,000 m^2) to arrive at a cost per m^2 of $20.69. The next step is to multiply the floor area of each department by the cost per m^2 to arrive at the indirect cost of estate management.

Table 4.4 Cost of estate management

Estates	Floor area (m^2)	Costs ($)
A&E	2 500	51 724
General medicine	4 000	82 759
Surgery	5 000	103 448
Renal	3 000	62 069
Paediatrics	4 500	93 103
Other	10 000	206 897
Total	29 000	600 000

The basis of apportionment

Apportionment across cost centres can be either:

- activity-based (e.g. the number of X-ray requests, number of operations); or
- non-activity-based (square metres, staff).

Activity-based costing involves looking at the actual activities within each cost centre and allocating costs so as to reflect a truer picture of the relative costs of different activities. So, in a pathology laboratory, for example, the costs would reflect not only the number of tests performed, but also the additional set-up and supervision costs of a rarely performed test. Another example would be an activity-based costing system that reflected the costs of specialist cleaning in an isolation ward (whereas traditional apportionment based on floor area would spread the cost across all wards in proportion to the floor area).

Whether to apply non-activity-based apportionment depends on the nature of the resource. You need to use non-activity-based apportionment when there is no meaningful measure of the workload provided for other cost centres. The basis can be, for example, space used, number of staff, total budgeted costs or some other alternative.

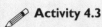

Activity 4.3

Match the following resources with the appropriate basis of apportionment:

1 Heating
2 CEO
3 Personnel officer
4 Pharmacist
5 Cleaning services

  a) total cost
  b) number of staff
  c) cubic metres
  d) number of requests
  e) square metres.

Feedback

1 (c), 2 (a), 3 (b), 4 (d), 5 (e)

These simple examples have shown that the way you categorize resources depends on the objective and the type of service that is being considered. In practice, shared costs may need to be treated in a more sophisticated way. A technical challenge of apportioning costs is to take into account service interdependencies. For example, services can be based on reciprocal arrangements. Housekeeping cleans the works departments and receives support from works. Apportionment can lead to different results depending on the basis that was used. This is a particular problem when the proportion of indirect costs and overheads is large as compared to direct costs, and for this reason activity-based costing is more often the preferred approach. Although the basis of apportionment won't change the total cost, it can be of concern for the manager whose services are subject to scrutiny. As a manager you will wish to ensure that costs that are being charged to your unit are calculated on a fair basis and that you are in a position to negotiate these if necessary.

Summary

There are two main purposes for recording costs depending on whether the information is to be used internally or externally. Management accounting aims to assist the day-to-day operation of a health care organization. Financial accounting is based on statutory requirements and aims to provide external bodies with accurate and true information regarding the organization's financial situation. A common way of analysing expenditure is to disaggregate spending into line items, functional costs and specialty costs. Financial coding systems can assist in this process. An alternative way of analysing cost is classification into direct costs, indirect costs and overheads. Indirect costs and overheads are costs of shared resources that need to be apportioned to the cost centre under consideration. The method of apportionment needs to be chosen carefully in order to avoid distortions between cost centres. Activity-based costing is designed to ensure that costs are shared in a way that more accurately reflects the actual costs of the activities associated with an identified cost object. In the next two chapters you will look at how this costing information is used to set prices.

5

Pricing decisions in health care

Overview

Pricing is one of the most critical decisions that an organization can make. In talking about pricing you will probably think about it as being something that impacts on whoever pays for the services provided. This is correct. But try to think about pricing more broadly too. Pricing is also an internal problem. Any time that costs are generated in one part of an organization a price needs to be agreed; that price is a cost to wherever it is transferred. The issues are still the same whether it is pricing internally to determine how much cost to transfer or externally to charge an appropriate amount for services provided. In this chapter you will examine the various pricing strategies and how they are reflected in decisions on service developments. When you have completed this chapter you will have an overview of the different objectives and methods of pricing which can be applied in the internal and external relations of an organization.

Learning objectives

By the end of this chapter you should be able to:

- **explain the objectives of pricing**
- **identify how these objectives are influenced by the laws of supply and demand**
- **apply marketing concepts such as the marketing mix and the Boston matrix to pricing decisions in health care markets**
- **describe different approaches to pricing**

Key terms

Absorption costing A costing approach recovering the average cost of a service.

Break-even activity level The activity level where total income equals total cost.

Internal pricing Charging for services between units of the same organization with the aim of increasing cost-consciousness and efficiency.

Marginal costing A costing approach recovering the variable cost of a service.

Marketing mix The mix of factors (price, product, place, promotion) to be controlled so that a service is provided in adequate quality and quantity.

Target pricing A pricing approach adding a mark-up to the cost per unit of service in order to make a profit.

Pricing

Economic theory suggests that the *price* regulates the quantity of a good or service demanded and supplied. Under perfect competition, firms are price-takers: they have little influence on pricing and have to accept the prices set by competitors for similar products. Under imperfect competition, firms are in control of prices as barriers to access, preventing competitors entering the market: think of a monopoly supplier of a new drug who is able to set prices at the desired level. But what about health care markets? These operate under imperfect conditions. The demand for health care is complicated because among other reasons it is based on need and often involves third-party payment. Consumer sovereignty is limited; decisions are often taken by health care professionals instead of the patients themselves.

Pricing in the private sector appears to be straightforward: a price is the money asked or paid for a service. For example, the price for a drug or a private practitioner's fee in an unregulated environment is subject to market forces. But how are prices set in the public sector? Usually third-party payment comes in and market forces are replaced by principles to achieve social goals. Public health agencies have a clear mission to purchase services that improve population health. With their pricing strategies they can encourage provision of health services that have characteristics of a public good and which therefore the private sector does not provide in sufficient quantities, such as health promotion, vector control or measures improving environmental health.

 ### Activity 5.1

From your experience of health services, give examples of pricing decisions of

1   Private providers.
2   Public providers.

 ### Feedback

1 Private sector prices are largely affected by market forces. In low-income countries with unregulated markets they depend essentially on local demand and supply. However, price discrimination in health care markets is not uncommon, if private providers have enough information as to who to charge higher prices. For example, for political reasons NGOs may charge more to the wealthy than to the poor. Usually there is also a segmentation of prices between rural and urban areas and between primary and secondary care. Fee schedules for private practitioners may exist in many countries but they are often not enforced by government. In countries where the private sector relies strongly on third-party buyers, pricing is regulated and subject to contractual arrangements.

2 As for the public sector, you will probably have thought of services provided free of charge because of the overall social benefit they provide, such as vaccination or health education. There is also a large range of services to which a price is attached, either in the form of charges to patients, such as user fees, or prices charged to third-party

payers (e.g. government or insurance companies). Think also of internal market arrangements where, under the overall umbrella of an organization, providers and purchasers negotiate prices for services.

Internal pricing

There are forms of *internal pricing* too. For example, under a policy of devolved clinical budgets clinicians may be charged for the laboratory tests they request which in turn may make them more selective about the requests they make. Systems of internal pricing are meant to increase cost-consciousness and efficiency. Any time that costs are generated in one part of an organization a price needs to be agreed; that price can then be charged to wherever the cost is transferred. Once you have established a price you can use it in many different ways. You can use this knowledge to analyse what your unit is being charged by other units and use this to negotiate the prices you are charged. In the same way, you can also use this to negotiate and justify the prices you want to pass on to other departments. Or, of course, you can apply this in establishing prices to charge external users of services or to justify requests for additional funding.

Prices and costs

Prices charged do not necessarily reflect full costs. For example, user fees tend to recover only a small percentage of total cost while, on the other hand, drug prices may contain a huge element of profit. Prices depend among other factors on the price of a substitute, the competition in the market-place and the value the consumer places on the product. For internal markets in most health systems there is a clear rule that total prices must equal total costs, as there is no way of recovering the surplus charged by any of the participants from the funding agency (Mellett *et al.* 1993).

What influences prices?

Pricing decisions in health services depend on a range of factors and are somewhat different from those taken in the commercial sector. In principle, whether a service is provided in an adequate way depends on the *marketing mix*, a concept that can easily be defined in terms of the four Ps:

* price;
* product;
* place;
* promotion.

Thus the price of a service depends on the quality of the service, the place where it can be obtained and the way it is made available to people. When analysing the marketing mix you will ask yourself in which ways certain characteristics of the service will affect pricing decisions and how customers (patients, third-party buyers or internal) perceive the balance between these categories (Pettinger 1994).

Product

Product describes the kind, quantity and quality of the service offered. Important criteria for health services are quality, diversity and timeliness of the service. You could charge more for services with a proven quality that cover a large range of treatment options and are available without undue delay. In a competitive environment pricing decisions are closely related to the market potential of each of the services offered. The relationship between market growth (in absolute terms) and market share (in relation to competitors) can be assessed quickly using the Boston Group matrix (Boston Consulting Group 1970) (see Figure 5.1).

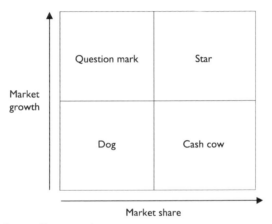

Figure 5.1 The Boston Group matrix

Managers need to know which of their services have a potential for growth or for achieving a higher market share. Take for example elective surgery in a department that can influence its service mix in response to market forces:

- *Cash cows:* these services are the main source of income of the department. They are produced in a high volume and low growth market. This could, for example, be the most frequently performed operations for which the hospital has a high expertise and market share.
- *Stars:* these services have the potential to become the main source of revenue in the future, though this may require a large investment to elaborate this position. For example, an operation based on a new method or technology which has not yet been adopted everywhere but which will potentially become the standard procedure in the future.
- *Question marks:* these services are problematic in terms of revenue. Even though they are part of a high growth market, the revenue gained by the service does not cover the investment required to increase the market share. Take, for

example, a new operation or technology that is offered by a nearby hospital with great expertise and sufficient funds to expand activity. You may not be able to keep up with your competitor and only a few providers will be able to offer this intervention in the future.

- *Dogs:* these services occupy a small market share with a low potential for growth, for example a niche market for special operations that are performed on a low number of patients. The service may be offered to maintain the reputation of the hospital, even though the generated revenue is low.

In publicly-funded systems where government regulates prices, providers have less scope for strategic portfolio decisions as service volumes and prices will depend on contracting. The key questions to be asked are whether the services offered meet the needs of the population and whether they can be provided with the desired quality and quantity. Purchasers may use pricing decisions to encourage or discourage provision of specific services. However, the relationship between market growth and market share remains important for regulating the provider mix. Government may set targets to achieve the participation of NGOs and private sector providers in the publicly-funded health care system.

Place

The location of the service may also affect pricing. Planning facilities at convenient locations with good transport could be a competitive advantage that allows higher prices to be charged. Likewise a hospital in an affluent urban area may charge higher prices than its counterpart in a rural region. The concept of place reflects the need for regional differentiation and responsiveness to customers' needs. Place is also strongly linked to achieving equity of access as a health care goal. However, there is a trade-off between decentralization and efficiency. Having too many decentralized units, for example one in each small town, will increase costs and prices per patient treated. Conversely, careful planning of geographical service expansion will contain costs and lead to lower prices. Decisions on place may also be driven by availability of staff if there is a lack of qualified staff on the labour market. Locations with a good infrastructure such as education facilities are more attractive to staff and this may also influence decisions on the location of a new service.

Promotion

This concept refers to the combination of methods used in the community to generate public awareness, confidence, acceptance and identification in relation to health services (Pettinger 1994). Lack of promotion may lead to underuse of services. Loss of confidence can be a challenge for managers and staff, where patients bypass local public services in favour of private services or more distant public services. Public health initiatives often require extensive promotion to be accepted. For example, a vaccination campaign may use methods of social marketing in order to achieve a higher coverage.

Consumers rely on word of mouth and seek information on the reputation of a provider. This is easy if there are only a few providers in a region, but with an increasing number of providers the available consumer information about each is limited. Thus promotion activities will increase with provider density. As advertising and marketing of health care is often limited by regulation, providers tend to 'signal' quality to consumers by the equipment they use and the qualifications of their staff (McPake *et al.* 2002).

Another important aspect of the marketing mix is *internal promotion* which seeks to increase the awareness of staff about the benefits of the service. When a new health programme is introduced, health workers need to be motivated and trained sufficiently in order to be able to gain trust and support from the community.

Activity 5.2

Use the dimensions of the marketing mix to analyse your organization. How do your customers (internal or external) perceive the services offered? In which ways are access to services in your organization influenced by price, product and place? Even if your organization has a fixed income with little influence on pricing, you still can consider the other dimensions of the marketing mix.

Feedback

Each of the components of the marketing mix may contribute in a unique way to important outcomes of the health service. A careful balance has to be maintained between each component and the other components. Price, promotion and place should all support the service being provided. All these affect the way a service is perceived and used. For high-quality services you would normally be able to charge a higher price. If services are offered at a low price then customers may think that they are of much lower quality than they really are. Likewise the way a service is promoted affects how it is perceived, as does the place where it is provided. The components of the marketing mix for your organization will be unique. Your answer should include a service definition or blueprint with established prices, a way of promoting the service and an explanation of the ways the place of delivery supports this.

Approaches to pricing

There are many objectives for pricing decisions but only two main approaches to pricing. One seeks to ensure that all costs are recovered and the other seeks to ensure that only the variable costs are recovered. The former is called *absorption costing*, the latter *marginal costing*. Both have a role to play.

- *Absorption costing* is intended to recover the full cost of providing services. This means that average costs are the basis of pricing. Overheads are fully apportioned to work out unit prices. The problem with this approach is that in a contractual environment, the planned activity must be met exactly to cover total costs. If activity deviates from the planned level, costs may be over- or under-recovered.
- *Marginal costing* is intended to recover the variable costs of providing services.

The problem with this approach is that a large proportion of the costs – the fixed costs – are not considered in pricing decisions.

Normally, private sector providers will add a mark-up to the costs in order to make a profit. This approach, which simply adds a percentage to the cost per unit of service, is called *target pricing*. Target pricing is less common in the public sector where price equals costs. Public sector providers may however be given the incentive to produce services at lower costs than projected and be permitted to retain the difference to the agreed price to improve service quality (Mellett *et al.* 1993).

If only the marginal costs are charged then customers should be getting outstanding value and demand for the service will be maximized. Such an approach is known as *penetration pricing* and is consistent with a cost-leadership strategy that attempts to maximize growth. The problem with penetration pricing is the persistent danger that fixed costs will not be covered. In practice, many organizations use a combination of both techniques: absorption costing for the bulk of services provided and marginal costing for negotiating new service developments. At the other extreme of pricing policies is *price skimming*: setting deliberately high prices to exploit a monopoly position. These examples show that choice of the costing method has a major impact on setting prices. In turn, pricing policy needs to reflect the strategic objectives of the organization.

Activity 5.3 Pricing and costing in your organization

Summarize the pricing policy for your organization and the costing methods on which it is based. Examine this both ways, looking at what happens outside the organization for users of the service, and look internally at what happens on recharges between departments.

Feedback

Most organizations use a combination of absorption and marginal costing approaches to price their services. If you are being charged for a service either by an external supplier or an internal department within your own organization, then you want to negotiate whether you should be charged on a marginal or a full cost basis. Marginal cost is more advantageous and if it is a full cost basis then you need to agree on the proportion of overheads that it is fair for you to be paying.

The relationship between income, expenditure and price

As you know there are different methods of paying health care providers, such as FFS, capitation payment and fixed budgets. Each creates different incentives influencing the behaviour of providers as to the quality and volume of the services provided. In the relationship between purchasers and providers there are three basic types of contract and each affects pricing behaviour in a specific way (England 2000). These are:

- block contracts;
- cost and volume contracts;
- cost per case.

Block contracts

Block contracts pay a fixed sum for a defined service. Take for example a primary care clinic that receives an annual lump sum for its services. Under this arrangement the income of the provider is cash-limited and if overspending occurs, the loss is usually covered by funds saved during the previous year. This is the simplest form of contract. The administrative costs are low and both purchaser and provider enjoy a high level of security as the contract is easy to manage and the financial risk is low. The price is usually based on the previous year's activity and the purchaser expects services of a similar kind and volume to be provided during the coming year. While block contracts can incorporate clauses for quality management and targets for outcomes of the service, they do not offer financial incentives to increase efficiency, neither by treating more patients nor by using fewer resources.

Cost and volume contracts

With *cost and volume contracts*, purchasers agree to pay a fixed price for a defined volume of services, for example for a specified number of patients or procedures. This type of contract adds a component of controlling activity, as additional payments or deductions can be agreed, if the actual quantity of services deviates from the agreed volume. For example, if the contracting parties agree on payment for 1000 cataract operations, additional operations may be paid at a different price. If purchasers intend to limit activity they will agree on setting a lower price for additional operations. If more activity is to be encouraged, higher prices will be set for additional cases. Obviously under this type of contract managers are challenged to control activity tightly. The contract should also ensure that all patients receive the appropriate quality of care. A drawback for providers is related to the risk of changes in morbidity. Costs may not be recovered fully if patients are sicker than anticipated and therefore use more resources. Reliable information on costs and activity is essential, which makes these contracts more complex and expensive to manage than simple block contracts. If the relevant information is available, cost and volume contracts can be used for providing health services in defined quantities that match community needs.

Cost per case

Cost per case contracts pay for each specific item of service. This could be, for example, an FFS arrangement where a practitioner or hospital receives a set fee from the insurance company for each patient treated. The number of cases treated is not limited and thus provider income increases with activity. Per case contracting can be considered if purchasers aim to increase provision of a certain type of service. Usually quality standards and overall targets for case numbers will be set. The approach is also useful for a small volume service. However, the administration and monitoring of cost per case contracts is costly as the purchaser is billed for each single patient. If per case contracting is used on a wide range of services and without limit to activity, services are likely to be produced in higher quantities than desired. Per case payment creates a strong incentive to increase income and may result in supplier-induced demand.

The three basic types of contract are often used in combination to achieve the desired provider behaviour. It is not unusual that providers have to oversee different types of contract with several purchasers and different prices.

While contracting is generally believed to improve access, efficiency and sustainability of service provision, the arrangements pose a challenge to managers. Contracts require careful monitoring, clear definitions of payment and perform-ance obligations and trust and willingness to avoid opportunistic behaviour. Both providers and purchasers must have the skills and capacity to manage contracts appropriately.

To be successful, the contracting process must achieve a balance between the interests of providers and purchasers. Purchasers need to be aware of the risk that providers may not be able to recover costs, if the contract is too tight. On the other hand they will try to avoid setting prices too high or creating perverse incentives that counteract the envisioned financial and public health goals.

Break-even analysis

For managers who are responsible for monitoring contracts, the break-even activity level is of special interest. This is the activity level where total income equals total cost. When activity increases beyond the break-even point the organization makes a surplus; if it stays below, the organization incurs a loss.

In Figure 5.2 the expenditure curve is combined with the total cost curve to allow for assessment of the break-even point. Under a cost per case contract the income curve starts at zero and increases steadily with activity. Break-even is achieved where income exceeds total costs. Under a block contract, the total cost curve would look similar but income would not change with activity and the income curve would run parallel to the x axis.

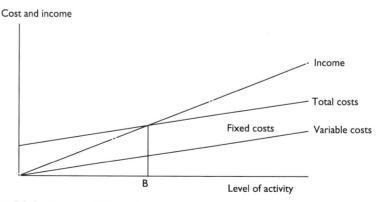

Figure 5.2 Break-even activity level

Activity 5.4

Describe the arrangements by which the income for your organization is paid. Is income paid on a lump-sum basis for a series of activities? Or is income paid for each activity you perform?

Feedback

If there is a block contract, then any additional services you perform may not be paid for. On the other hand, the payment of a lump sum for a block contract can give a lot of certainty to plan ahead and security for the future. In a cost per case scenario it may be difficult to recover total cost, as the example of the laboratory has shown in Chapter 2. But it also offers the opportunity to produce a surplus as activity increases. So do cost and volume contracts if there are provisions for additional payment when the activity exceeds the agreed target.

Summary

A price is the money asked or paid for a service. As internal markets are based on a cash-limited system, total prices must equal total costs. In making pricing decisions a careful balance has to be maintained between each component of the marketing mix (price, product, place and promotion). Pricing policies reflect the strategic goals of an organization. They can vary to the extent that they aim to recover costs. Most organizations use a combination of absorption and marginal costing approaches to price their services. You looked at three basic types of contract between purchasers and providers of health care that affect provider behaviour in a specific way: block, cost and volume and cost per case.

References

Boston Consulting Group (1970) *The Product Portfolio*. Boston, MA: BCG Publications.

England, R. (2000) *Contracting and Performance Management in the Health Sector: Some Pointers on How to Do It*. London: Department for International Development (DFID) Health Systems Resource Centre.

McPake, B., Kumaranayake, L. and Normand, C. (2002) *Health Economics: An International Perspective*. London: Routledge.

Mellett, H., Marriott, N. and Harries, S. (1993) *Financial Management in the NHS: A Manager's Handbook*. London: Chapman & Hall.

Pettinger, R. (1994) *Introduction to Management*. London: Macmillan.

6 | The pricing process in different settings

Overview

In this chapter you will look at practical examples of managing prices: setting user fees and various forms of contract pricing. The chapter also reviews the two main approaches to costing: the bottom-up approach and the top-down approach. The former entails a detailed costing of all the components of a service, which is very time-consuming and expensive. The latter entails a more broad-brush estimate of the cost of services – this may be less accurate, but it is easier to perform. Both approaches have an important role to play.

Learning objectives

By the end of this chapter you should be able to:

- **describe ways of setting user fees for health services**
- **explain approaches to pricing under different contractual arrangements**
- **describe the use of DRGs in pricing and discuss the advantages and limitations of this approach**
- **explain the bottom-up and the top-down approaches to costing**

Key terms

Base rate The average cost across all DRGs. Base rates are not only calculated for individual hospitals but also to compare cost per case across a region or the entire country.

Bottom-up costing A detailed approach identifying the costs of all inputs.

Case-mix index A measure of disease severity across all cases treated in an entire department or hospital during a year, usually calculated as the sum of all relative costs weights divided by the number of cases.

Cost weight A factor reflecting the relative cost of a single diagnosis related group DRG. By definition the cost weight of the base rate is 1.0, DRGs with a resource use below average have a cost weight < 1, above average of >1.

Diagnosis related group (DRG) Classification system that assigns patients to categories on the basis of the likely cost of their episode of hospital care. Used as basis for determining level of prospective payment by purchaser.

DRG creep (upcoding) A form of DRG misclassification leading to unjustified high reimbursement levels.

> **Prospective payment** Paying providers before any care delivered based on predefined activity levels and anticipated cost.
>
> **Top-down costing** An approach based on average costs.
>
> **Unit of activity (currency)** The unit used to measure the activity, such as operations, bed days or laboratory tests.

Setting user fees

As you saw in the previous chapter, pricing is important for all organizations. Even if the government pays for everything, identifying some form of prices for your services can help you justify your funding and get more money to support your activities. A critical decision is whether to charge user fees for health services. Charging clients can mobilize some additional revenue but it may also deter potential users.

Once a decision on user fees has been reached, practical management problems need to be resolved:

- how to set the fee level;
- how to collect money;
- how to set up a system of financial controls;
- what exemptions and waivers should apply.

User fees may be charged for a variety of purposes. The additional revenue could be used to improve the quality of services, make an organization less reliant on donor or government, or even be a matter of survival where client charges are the only source of income. If fees constitute only a small proportion of total income, the costs of fee collection and financial control may be too high relative to the revenue collected. It is therefore important to implement a system that is easy to use and that requires minimal additional work for staff.

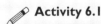 **Activity 6.1**

Read the following summary, prepared from 'Charging fees for family planning services' (Management Sciences for Health 1992) about charging fees for family planning services. Focus on the issues related to the different forms that user fees can take and consider the requirements for administration and financial control needed by each of them. Assume you have to recover a large proportion of cost through client charges. Consider the relative advantages and disadvantages of the different forms the fee can take.

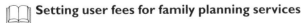 **Setting user fees for family planning services**

Family planning services are frequently co-financed through client fees and the sale of products to clients or other organisations. The idea behind this is that clients who pay a fee are more likely to value the services they receive. It enables them to demand high quality services. It has also been shown that clients who pay for contraceptives are more likely to use them.

However, the cost of implementing a system of service charges should always be less than the projected income from the fees. The system should be easy to administer and require minimal additional work for clinic staff. An accurate estimate of the costs of each service will assist the clinic to justify the level at which to set the fee and to determine how much of the costs can be reasonably recovered. Most of the revenue generated should be used at the clinic's discretion to support its own activities, such as improving the services or the facility. Part of the fees can also be used to increase financial self-sufficiency of the organisation and expand its services to specific populations of clients in a poor or underserved area.

There are a number of different types of fees some of which can combined:

- Registration fees are a set amount collected from the client at each visit.
- Membership fees charge clients a fixed amount on a yearly basis, entitling them to a range of clinic services.
- Service fees are charged for each service provided, for example for examination, laboratory tests or counselling.
- Fees for contraceptives can be charged separately from other services clients receive.

When deciding on how much to charge, the organisation could either perform a survey on what clients are able and willing to pay or set a fee based on what clients pay for services at other family planning or health care facilities. Another way is to set the fees in line with the price of common household commodities, such as a kilo of rice, a litre of oil, or a soft drink. In one health zone in Zaire, managers decided that the price of a monthly membership fee should not exceed the price of two kilos of soybeans. An alternative approach for setting fee levels is to establish specific cost recovery objectives. An organisation may wish to recover 20% of its operating costs in order to be able to expand services to the poor or open a new facility.

The administrative costs of implementing user fees must be considered from early on. A supervisory system should be in place to ensure accuracy and avoid misuse. A basic system of controls should incorporate the processes of collecting fees, cash handling, and accounting for income and expenses. Information from the activity register with records of the services provided and the contraceptives dispensed should be compared regularly with the collected charges, to make sure that all financial transactions are recorded correctly.

A system for waiving or reducing fees should be decided to enable access of the poor to the service. Such a system should be made administratively simple and have controls to ensure that it is not abused. A simple questionnaire can help assess the client's economic status and charges may be set on a sliding-fee scale based on household income and family size. The mode of payment should be flexible, so that clients who cannot afford the fee, may pay in kind.

Finally it is essential to inform the community about the new fee structure with its exemptions, waivers, price reductions, or payment options and explain that the income from the fees is being used to improve service quality and to subsidise the cost of providing services for people who are unable to pay.

Feedback

Membership and registration fees have the advantage that clients are charged a fixed amount per year or per visit, entitling them to a range of clinic services. Note that the annual membership fee is similar to a simple prepaid insurance scheme. Fee collection is easy to administer and gives providers some security in planning. A potential disadvantage could be that individual users may consume more services than are covered by the fee. In contrast, service fees are charged for each service provided but involve higher levels of skills of financial control and administration. Thus the costs of establishing and operating fee collection are relatively high. Furthermore, the provider bears a risk if fewer services are paid for than planned. Often fees for contraceptives are charged separately from other services clients receive. Depending on the set price, this approach can be used to direct clients to lower cost sources, for example pharmacies, while the facility concentrates on clinical methods and counselling.

Generally user fees will recover part of the costs and free up resources to expand the availability of services. They may also lessen dependence on government or donor funds. However, price increases may have a strong impact on demand and dissuade clients from using the service. Effective mechanisms must be in place to ensure that the poor have access to the service.

Contract pricing

The problem of matching income with prices is more complicated in a contractual environment, where the total cost needs to be recovered by the prices at which services are purchased. Many countries use service contracts to arrange payment of health care providers. These can be one-year contracts, though more commonly three- to five-year commissioning agreements are being used, which then are effectively long-term contracts. Whatever the time period and however the service is specified in a commissioning agreement, there is a need to have an overview of what services are provided and what these are worth. Pricing is closely related to the planning of future expenditure (budgeting), as you will see in the next chapter. For hospital financing there are two basic forms of payment: retrospective and prospective reimbursement.

- In a *retrospective reimbursement* system the hospital sets a price that covers the full cost incurred during the previous year regardless of activity. This method has been abandoned in many countries. It is inefficient as it discourages cost containment (Donaldson and Gerard 1993).
- In a *prospective reimbursement* system prices are calculated for a defined activity level. Payment can take different forms. Contracts with funding agencies can be agreed for a pre-defined budget that reflects the demanded level of activity. In acute care this is usually treatment of a defined number of cases, and in long-term care the number of bed-days can be used. The agreements need to include provision for the volume of activity anticipated and provision for what should happen if activities are higher or lower than planned. Or DRGs can be used to identify patient groups with similar resource use, in which case prices are prospectively set according to the average cost for each DRG. Here the number of cases can be agreed or left to the discretion of the hospital. All methods produce

specific adverse incentives and they are usually combined with additional measures to increase efficiency.

The first stage in pricing is to identify and define the product or service you are pricing. Whatever is defined as the service can be used to measure the activities delivered. This could be the number of cases, bed-days, lab tests or operations performed. This is referred to as either the *unit of activity* or contract *currency*. This can be used to negotiate, measure and manage activity.

✎ Activity 6.2

Under a prospectively fixed budget, which unit of activity could be used for:

1 Acute care.
2 Long-term nursing care.

↻ Feedback

In acute care, a purchaser would agree on the number of cases to give providers incentives to use resources efficiently and to minimize length of stay (LOS). This could be the overall number of patients per year or the number of operations performed, or you could define cases according to DRGs. Case definition in health care is complicated because of the wide range of different conditions that patients can have and the wide range of treatments that can be applied. The least likely unit of activity you would use is the number of occupied hospital beds. This gives providers a strong incentive to increase LOS as it did when retrospective reimbursement was common in many countries. This explains in part the large international variation in LOS between countries which use different reimbursement systems.

In contrast, long-term care activity is usually measured in days of care (or bed days). The number of days of care is limited by the number of available places the institution offers and the occupancy level. Because there is little variation in resource use over time, occupancy is of more concern for efficient resource use than LOS. Similar pricing arrangements on cost per day can be found in day care for the elderly, palliative care, or in homes for people with learning disabilities. Different price levels or extra charges can be agreed according to different levels of medical and nursing needs.

If the unit of activity is bed-days, you can easily work out the cost per day if you know total costs and occupancy. In the following example a facility of 50 beds is run with an occupancy of 95 per cent. Occupancy is calculated as (days of care/bed-days available) × 100.

	US$
Fixed costs	1,500,000
Variable costs	500,000
Total costs	2,000,000

Number of places: 50

Days of care available: 50×365 18,250

Days of care at 95% occupancy: 17,338

Cost per day: 2,000,000/17,338   US$115

If the price charged is the cost per day, the provider will run into a deficit if the expected occupancy is not achieved, as fixed costs are under-recovered. As you will see in the next activity, in a case-based pricing system a similar problem might arise, if the actual number of cases treated is smaller than projected.

Activity 6.3

A hospital department has agreed to perform 500 eye operations at a price of $4000 per case. The price calculation was based on the anticipated costs as shown below. During the year it turns out that demand has declined and only 450 patients could be treated. Work out costs per case for treating 450 cases by completing the calculations using the data given.

Anticipated costs for 500 patients		*Cost/case*
Fixed costs	1,500,000	3,000
Variable costs	500,000	1,000
Total costs	**2,000,000**	**4,000**

Actual costs for 450 patients:
Fixed costs:
Variable costs:
Total costs:

Feedback

You will have found that the department will make a loss of $333 per case, as part of the fixed costs is not recovered. This loss is much higher ($450 \times \$333.3 = 150,000$) than the savings of variable costs due to the reduced case number.

Anticipated costs for 500 patients		*Cost/case*
Fixed costs	1,500,000	3,000
Variable costs	500,000	1,000
Total costs	**2,000,000**	**4,000**

Actual costs for 450 patients:		
Fixed costs	1,500,000	3,333
Variable costs	450,000	1,000
Total costs	**1,950,000**	**4,333**

In health services most costs are fixed costs rather than variable costs, so the major influence on pricing is going to be what assumptions are made for the anticipated volumes of activity. For example, if most of the costs are fixed then if the volume of activity doubles, the average cost will approximately halve.

Alternatively, if most costs are fixed and the volume of activity halves, the average cost will approximately double. This can be a major factor for deficits. If the actual activity is less than anticipated then not all of the fixed costs will be recovered and a deficit will occur.

So usually the contracting parties will agree on contingencies to share the risk if the case number is higher or lower than agreed.

Using DRGs as a pricing system

In the last decade DRGs have become increasingly popular as a prospective payment for hospital services. A DRG allows a fixed price to be set for all cases of the same diagnostic category. Purchasers can set the reimbursement level to the average cost for each DRG and the hospital is usually free to decide on the number of cases treated, the inputs used and length of stay.

Under this system providers have strong incentives to increase efficiency by offering services at near to or below average price (Donaldson and Gerard 1993). Hospitals will for example make a surplus by delivering the service with a shorter LOS, by specializing in certain treatments, by substituting inputs or achieving economies of scale by treating large number of cases.

Calculating prices for different DRGs is made easy by use of *cost weights*. Every DRG is linked to a cost weight which reflects the resource use according to disease severity and the complexity of the procedures employed. Usually the average cost across all DRGs is chosen as a reference value, which is called the *base rate*. For example, if the base rate is $2000 (an arbitrary number) and the actual average cost for treating a case with a specific disease is $4000, then a cost weight of 2.0 will be attached to this DRG, as the cost of treatment is double the cost of an average case. Thus, by definition the cost weight of the base rate is 1.0, DRGs with a resource use below average have a cost weight < 1, above average of >1.

The cost weight takes account of the actual input needed for treating a case. For example, a complicated case of appendicitis will attract a relatively high cost weight of 2.02, to reflect the longer hospital stay after the appendectomy. The income/price (I) for this case would be:

Cost weight × base rate = I

$2.02 \times \$2000 \quad = \$4040$

In contrast, if the cost weight for an uncomplicated appendicitis is 1.09, the hospital would receive only 1.09 × $2000 = $2180.

Base rates are not only calculated for individual hospitals but also to compare cost per case across a region or the entire country. The *regional base rate* is an important comparator in a competitive environment which can be used by purchasers to set prices. Providers whose internal base rate is below the regional average will have a competitive advantage, those with a base rate higher than the regional average will make a loss.

Monitoring case mix

Internationally, DRG systems and approaches to monitoring case mix vary widely. Some countries use only 20 DRGs, others more than 800. To be able to negotiate prices, managers need excellent information about the costs and case mix of the services provided. A tool that is frequently used for this is the *case-mix index* (CMI).

The CMI is an average measure of disease severity across all cases treated in an entire department or hospital during a year. Take for example a department with only two types of DRG: 100 cases were treated with a relative weight of 2.02, and 50 cases with a relative weight of 1.09, and the CMI is:

$(100 \times 2.02) + (50 \times 1.09) = 256.5$ which is to be divided by the total number of 150 cases: $256.5/150 = 1.71$

As a department will have many more than just two types of case, the calculation is applied in an analogous way to all DRGs used in the department. The CMI expresses average disease severity of all cases treated by the department and allows annual income to be assessed quickly, provided all cases are coded properly and assigned to the correct DRG. Similarly, the departmental CMIs can be combined to create one CMI for the entire hospital:

Income from DRGs = number of cases × CMI × base rate

Case classification and calculation of the CMI is usually assisted by information systems, which will support the analysis of both the number and types of patients treated, and the mix of treatments and procedures provided.

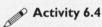 **Activity 6.4**

Assume a hospital operates four departments with the following CMI and number of cases.

Table 6.1 Hospital case mix data

Department	CMI	Number of cases	DRG-related income
A	1.2	2 800	
B	0.9	4 000	
C	2.3	900	
D	1.4	2 000	
Entire hospital		9 700	
Hospital base rate	2 000		
Regional base rate	1 800		
Expected loss			

1 Work out the DRG-related income on the basis of an internal base rate of $2000.
2 The expected regional base rate that purchasers are prepared to pay is $1800. Which strategies could the hospital use to avoid making a loss during the coming year?

Feedback

The completed table should look like this:

Table 6.2 DRG-related income

Department	CMI	Number of cases	DRG-related income
A	1.2	2 800	6 720 000
B	0.9	4 000	7 200 000
C	2.3	900	4 140 000
D	1.4	2 000	5 600 000
Entire hospital	1.219	9 700	23 660 000
Hospital base rate			
Regional base rate	1 800		21 294 000
Expected loss			2 366 000

The CMI for the entire hospital is approximately 1.219. The difference between the internal and the regional base rate is $200, indicating that the hospital's competitors treat patients more cheaply and are thus able to offer their services at a lower price. In order to avoid a loss of $2.3 million the hospital should review its services and use fewer resources on those cases where costs exceed the regional average. It could also try to increase the number of cases where it achieves a surplus. Just increasing the number of cases or treating more severe cases to increase the CMI without improving the cost structure would not be sufficient.

As the example shows, DRG systems can offer strong incentives to use resources efficiently. However, the approach to pricing can also be linked to serious negative effects, particularly when DRGs are not specific enough to reflect the complexity of a case and thus the correct level of resource use. Using DRGs is rather complex and expensive because it involves good information about the costs per case and careful monitoring of the case mix.

Activity 6.5

Take some time and reflect on the above example from a purchaser's point of view. Think of the different forms of inappropriate provider behaviour which may occur in relation to quality and quantity of the service provision under a DRG system. What measures could be taken to avoid these?

Feedback

Pricing systems based on DRGs will usually make a range of provisions to discourage unwanted provider behaviour. As in any other case-based payment system the quality of the service may suffer if providers try to cut corners. This is usually addressed by rigorous internal and external audit and specifically designed programmes of quality assurance.

Providers may also prefer to treat only those cases where they can easily recover costs or make a surplus. This may lead to underprovision of services and inappropriate admissions and discharge. Underprovision can arise when expected case numbers are small and thus relatively expensive to treat. This may occur in remote and rural areas. Additional incentives are usually given to run hospitals in such areas.

Inappropriate admissions and early discharge are problems where competition is strong. This may occur when the provider expects that the costs of a specific case are under-recovered. The more extreme effects are known as:

• cost shifting, i.e. shifting costs onto other sectors of care or
• patient shifting, i.e. referring patients to other providers

Providers could also try to increase case numbers by readmitting the same patient several times for short episodes of care. To avoid this kind of behaviour, the price per DRG can be differentiated according to LOS. The full price is paid if the case is treated within the set range of days, a slightly lower amount is paid if patients need to stay longer, and a much lower price (or nothing) is paid if LOS falls below the set minimum.

The second set of challenges is related to coding of cases. You would expect that hospitals will use the patient classification system in their best interest to achieve the highest possible price for each case. Because disease severity, complications and comorbidity are all factors which attract higher cost weights, providers will tend to keep the CMI at a high level. Inappropriate coding of cases, inadvertently or deliberately, is not uncommon and patients may thereby appear sicker than they are. This form of misclassification, which is called *DRG creep* or *upcoding*, leads to unjustified reimbursement levels. In response purchasers will monitor changes of the CMI carefully and review records of selected cases. Also, DRGs should be updated yearly to reflect changes in medical practice or the introduction of new technologies as accurately as possible (Nowicki 2001).

Practical approaches to pricing

All the settings you have considered so far require a sound knowledge of the costs. If detailed information is available on all the steps required to treat a patient, then it is possible to do a highly detailed bottom-up costing, and cost every aspect of the service. So you would identify the costs of all inputs such as costs of staff, technical and medical supplies, consumables, overheads for administration, maintenance, energy costs, facility management and capital costs.

If, however, this detailed information is not available then a top-down approach to costing is the only method that can be used, and prices are based on the cost of treating the average patient, based in turn on the number of patients treated. In practice, because health care is such a complicated service, both methods are used: highly detailed, bottom-up costing for conditions that occur frequently and are predictable, and averaging for the remaining, less predictable and less frequently occurring patient conditions using the top-down approach.

Note that there are also differences in the cost and feasibility between the two approaches (Mellett *et al.* 1993).

- The *bottom-up approach* is expensive and time-consuming to calculate as it depends on accurate treatment profiles and identification of resources used, and then costing this accurately. The advantage is that the costings tie in with clinical practice so that clinicians find these helpful in trying to manage financial performance. As clinical practice changes, so too these costings will change.
- The *top-down method* of costing is quick and easy to calculate but there is no linkage to variation in clinical practice as it is based on average costs. It is suitable for low-volume, low-cost procedures.

Both approaches can also be combined in different ways. For example, to work out the costs of chronic dialysis for patients with end-stage renal failure, you could first do a detailed bottom-up appraisal for the technical inputs of dialysis. In a second step you could estimate human resource costs in a top-down approach, by separating the staff costs and overheads for chronic dialysis from those of the other activities of the department, such as acute dialysis, the renal ward and transplantation services. Or in a chain of health centres with a similar cost structure you could perform a detailed bottom-up approach to identify the costs of one specific service, for example detection and treatment of TB cases, and apply the findings in a top-down approach to the other centres.

Stages in the costing and pricing process

As you have seen from the case studies and examples presented, costing and pricing are closely related and the process for both needs to be planned carefully. To participate in costing and pricing, or perhaps even introduce it in your own organization, you need to have a view of the stages involved, both to know where and how to contribute to your existing costing and pricing processes, and to design new ones.

1 Define clearly the service for which you want to calculate prices (e.g. malaria case detection and treatment, renal replacement therapy, psychiatric day clinic). Define the unit of activity or 'currency' you want to use to set prices.
2 Identify the costs of providing this service, using either a top-down or bottom-up approach as discussed above.
3 Decide on the level of costs you aim to recover by pricing. This could be either average costs or marginal costs. Pricing decisions will vary widely with the objectives of the provider and market conditions. User fees may cover only a small proportion of costs, whereas private sector prices will try to cover costs plus a profit margin.
4 Take account of the planned activity level. This is likely to be the most difficult part of the exercise.
5 Account for any associated costs (e.g. costs of training, research or teaching). This depends on whether these costs should be included in the price of the service or be reimbursed separately.
6 Adjust for inflation. This can be a major problem in countries with high inflation rates. Instead of using an average rate use different rates for staff, energy, drugs, etc., if available.
7 Work out the price per unit of activity.

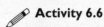 **Activity 6.6**

Now relate the stages in the costing and pricing process to what happens in your own organization.

1 Identify the services for which prices are calculated.
2 What activity data are available? What improvements could be made to the workload/activity data?
3 What costing methods are applied?
4 How is activity level taken into account?

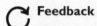 **Feedback**

Your organization will have its own unique approach to costing and pricing. You will have found ways of improving the pricing process. In completing this exercise you should not feel yourself restricted by what your organization actually does. If you feel there is a better way that things should be done, then why not list this instead? What is important is that you think critically and constructively about what actually happens and what is needed or could be done. You may have listed the basic forms of contract that apply to your organization, such as block, cost and volume and cost per case contracts. The approach to costing may be based on a bottom-up or a top-down approach or a combination of both. Target pricing may occur in the private sector. It is also not uncommon to compare your prices with the market leader, though this clearly requires some knowledge of what your competitors include in their prices. Costing software is frequently used to improve consistency. If a DRG system is used, the quality of coding is very important. In order to increase accuracy, professional coders can be used to support clinical staff in the correct use of the patient classification system.

Summary

Pricing is of practical interest in many different areas of health services. You looked at setting user fees for a family planning service and at pricing methods in a contractual relationship between health care purchasers and providers. In the hospital sector, DRGs are increasingly used to reimburse providers and you learned how this approach works, how regional base rates can be used to compare prices between hospitals and in which ways inappropriate provider behaviour in setting prices can be controlled. The chapter has described the different stages of defining the service, identifying costs and adjusting for inflation. As most costs are fixed rather than variable in health services, pricing is largely influenced by the planned volumes of activity. In assessing costs, two methods can be used: a highly detailed, bottom-up approach for services that occur frequently and are predictable, and a top-down approach for less frequent and less predictable services.

References

Donaldson, C. and Gerard, K. (1993) *Economics of Health Care Financing: The Visible Hand*. London: Macmillan.

Management Sciences for Health (1992) Charging fees for family planning services, *The Family Planning Manager*, 1(3): 1–12.

Mellett, H., Marriott, N. and Harries, S. (1993) *Financial Management in the NHS: A Manager's Handbook*. London: Chapman & Hall.

Nowicki, M. (2001) *The Financial Management of Hospitals and Healthcare Organizations*, 2nd edn. Chicago: Health Administration Press.

7 | Budgets and budgeting techniques

Overview

As a manager you are accountable for the financial performance of the activities under your control. Unless you can justify how you are spending the money allocated to you in your budget, you are vulnerable to the potentially unjustified criticism of others and will always struggle to keep hold of the financial resources already allocated to you, or to secure additional resources for your unit. The skills needed for budgeting are easy to learn and to apply.

Learning objectives

After working through this chapter you should be able to:

- **examine your departmental budget and identify the key features**
- **explain some motivational and behavioural aspects of budgeting**
- **describe different approaches to budgeting and compare the advantages and disadvantages of these**
- **analyse budget variances into volume and price components**
- **use variance analysis to identify the underlying causes of variances**

Key terms

Budget A tool for relating planned resource consumption to a period of time.

Cost variance A variance that arises because the cost of resources was greater or lower than anticipated.

Efficiency variance A variance that arises because the labour input or the cost of overheads was higher or lower than planned.

Flexible budgeting Systems designed to allow budgets to respond to changes in workload and activity as the budget period progresses.

Incremental budgeting An approach which involves taking the previous period's budget and adjusting the figures to reflect the changes in planned activity levels and in costs and prices for the forthcoming year.

Profiling The technique used to adjust for seasonal variations within a budget, so that actual progress can be monitored against the budget.

Usage variance A variance that arises because the volume of resources used was higher or lower than planned.

Variance The difference between planned and actual activity.

Zero-based budgeting A budgeting method that identifies and costs all of the inputs that will be required to achieve the desired level of activity and outcome.

What is a budget?

A *budget* can be defined as 'a tool used to relate planned resource consumption to a period of time' (Mellett *et al.* 1993). This definition highlights the three main features of a budget:

- it is a plan that is developed before an event has occurred;
- it can include a broad range of resources – not just money;
- it relates to a specific period of time.

Budgets are used at many levels in health care, from the national down to the level of provider units. The exact levels and ways in which budgets are determined will depend on the financing system in operation in the country concerned.

The role of budgets within the planning framework

As you saw briefly in Chapter 2, budgets have a particular role to play within the overall strategic planning framework of an organization. Figure 7.1 presents this framework for a typical health service organization. Senior managers engage in long-term planning, agreeing high-level objectives and identifying programmes or levels of service delivery that will enable them to meet these objectives. Then, by calculating the costs and benefits of alternative programmes and of alternative combinations of services, senior and middle managers are able to come to decisions as to the strategy they will adopt. A set of budgets is constructed to translate the strategic objectives into detailed operational plans. A budget for a hospital, for example, will be made up of budgets for each of the different operational units, combined to make up department budgets which are in turn collated with the income budget to form a master budget for the hospital.

The different types of budget and the ways in which they are constructed will be described in Chapter 8. In this chapter the focus is on typical departmental budgets.

Budgets enable managers to identify the resources that will be needed to achieve target levels of activity or desired outcomes. Budgets also serve a number of other purposes. Drury (1996) lists the reasons for producing budgets as:

1 To aid the planning of annual operations.
2 To coordinate the activities of the various parts of the organization and to ensure that the parts are in harmony with each other.
3 To communicate plans to the various responsibility centre managers.
4 To motivate managers to strive to achieve the organizational goals.
5 To control activities.
6 To evaluate the performance of managers.

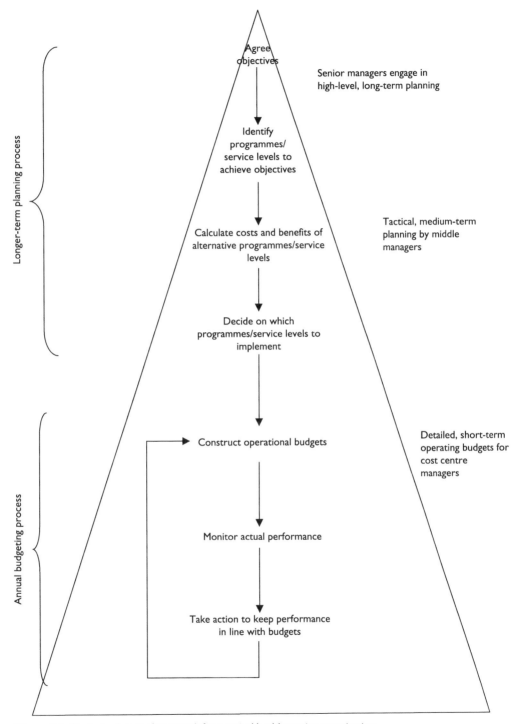

Figure 7.1 Strategic planning framework for a typical health service organization

A budget, once agreed and implemented, is then used to monitor actual activity and expenditure against the levels set out in the budget and to analyse the differences (known as *variances*) between planned and actual activity. So a budget is both a planning and a control tool and is essential to the management of organizations.

It follows from the above that the benefits of budgeting are that it:

- facilitates the control of resources;
- allows managers to assess performance;
- identifies the extent to which individual managers can contribute to achieving the objectives of the organization;
- provides early warning of variations from plans.

Devolving budgets

Budgets are the central link between planning and control. They are quantitative statements which allow agreed financial and policy objectives to be pursued for a set period of time. Projected income is the basis for planning expenditure, which can be traced down with an increasing level of detail from the entire organization to departments, units and eventually individual patients. Different ways of analysing spending and the corresponding types of budget can be found within a single organization. They are used in a sequence of steps in devolving a centrally administered budget to organizational units (Mellett *et al.* 1993; Cook 1995).

1 The budgeting process starts with identifying the financial inputs of the organization.
2 The total financial input is analysed by basic categories of expenditure for staff, goods and services. Each line item can be further subdivided, for example salaries for doctors and nurses, supplies, equipment and services obtained from outside the organization if applicable, such as cleaning or catering. This way of looking at expenditure is sometimes called *subjective analysis*.
3 In a next step funds can be analysed by objectives of the service (*objective analysis*). The central budget can be devolved to the functions of the organization, for example, horizontal or vertical programmes, primary or secondary care or clinical departments of a hospital. Within an organization or programme, expenditure on administration, energy, facility management and other items that are shared by all units is considered as overheads. Overheads can be apportioned to the units according to the resources they consume. Devolved budgets are commonly used where central government entrusts funds to the regional and district level. In large hospitals, devolved clinical budgets can be used in a similar way, with managers being responsible for each unit.
4 Finally, expenditure can be analysed by type of patient care. At the clinical level a range of further analyses is possible, for example, looking at inpatient or outpatient treatment, clinical specialty (orthopaedics, general surgery etc), disease categories for case-based reimbursement (DRGs) and even individual expenditure profiles, assessing the resource use of patient X or Y.

Activity 7.1

Why are devolved budgets so popular? Certainly they are a means of increasing the accountability of management and increasing flexibility in response to local needs. More specifically, according to Garbutt (1992), devolved budgets help managers to:

a) allocate resources
b) quantify plans
c) coordinate unit activities
d) communicate management plans and objectives
e) set performance objectives and targets
f) plan and control business performance

Think for a while whether these goals are met in your organization.

1 If your organization has devolved budgets, investigate how these are managed and whether all six objectives are achieved in the context of your organization. First review your unit's budget and identify the key features. Look at the layout, the income and cost items reported. To check that you have identified the key features, review how your budget achieves the six objectives of devolved budgets mentioned above.

2 If your organization does not have devolved budgets, then use this activity to make a case for budgets to be devolved to the unit level, stating how devolved budgets would help the unit manager in achieving these goals.

Feedback

1 Every unit will be different. While objectives (a) to (c) are straightforward and certainly supported by devolved budgets, objectives (d) to (f) are more difficult to achieve as they require that clinicians are held responsible for the decisions they make (Cook 1995). You need to consider how clinical performance targets can be achieved for your unit and whether these can be integrated more closely with your unit budget if they are not close. Each clinical decision, for example prescribing a drug, implies a financial decision on resource use. Also, strategic and operational planning makes no sense if the objectives are not agreed with the clinical staff responsible for the department. Therefore, activity levels need to be planned together with the relevant clinical staff and, increasingly, clinical pathways and guidelines are used to reduce variation of the financial impact of clinical decisions.

2 Were you able to make a strong case for devolved budgeting? Or would you argue that in your unit, as in many health service units, it is difficult to agree on fundamental objectives to be set in clinical terms and that for this reason devolved budgets would be unlikely to contribute to achieving objectives (d) to (f)?

With devolution of responsibility within health care, units are being given increasing responsibility for their own budgets. As you have seen, these are referred to as cost centres. It is important that a unit has clearly defined boundaries so that managers are aware of the extent of their responsibilities for resources. Units often trade with each other for the provision of services and this system allows them to compare the cost of services provided by internal providers with those of services that could be bought in.

A unit budget

An example of a budget for a health care unit is set out in Table 7.1. This budget shows only the amounts that the unit plans to spend in providing services during the year beginning 1 April 2005. To arrive at these figures, however, the budget manager would need to begin by specifying the *level* of services to be provided.

Table 7.1 Annual budget for a health care unit

Budget heading	Budgeted expenditure 1.4.05 to 31.3.06 (US$)
Nursing costs	3 019 148
Medical equipment costs	104 980
Medical staff costs	767 220
Management costs	300 778
Consumables	342 466
Administration costs	194 724
Total	4 729 316

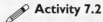 **Activity 7.2**

Suggest how the activities of the following services might be specified for budgeting purposes.

1 A hospital ward.
2 A family planning clinic.
3 A radiology unit.
4 A physiotherapy department.

 Feedback

For some of these services there may be several possible measures of activity. Did you suggest measures such as the following?

1 Bed-days, calculated as the number of beds in a ward times the number of days the ward is open.

2 The number of clients seen.

3 The number of X-rays produced.

4 The number of treatments supplied.

A budget is a list of all the inputs required to reach the planned activity levels for the year. These are usually organized into headings classifying the different types of input. Thus if you were providing acute hospital services you might classify inputs as:

1 Those related to patient care, including medical and nursing staff, drugs, theatre time, pathology, pharmacy, occupational therapy and radiography.
2 General services, including catering, domestics, portering, medical records, administration and estate management.

The budget package should also include details of the extent of the freedom to manipulate resources within the total budget. For example, to what extent could a manager use savings from the drugs budget to pay for an additional staff post?

Motivational and behavioural implications of budgeting

Budgets have significant motivational and behavioural implications. Giving responsibility for budgets can be a way of delegating that leaves it up to the manager to get on with the day-to-day activities so long as the targets in the budget are achieved. However, when budgets are imposed on managers who have had little or no influence over their construction, they may be viewed as restrictive and the manager may not be motivated to achieve the outcomes specified in the budget. In all organizations it is essential that those who are to be held responsible for a budget are actively involved in setting that budget.

The challenges in health services

In health services there is a potential conflict between clinicians who make the spending decisions and managers who are responsible for keeping costs at budgeted levels. It is important that clinicians and managers work together to identify and agree resourcing priorities, or that clinicians take on the management role.

Another concern is that managers who are responsible for a cost centre but who are not in a position to influence activity (and therefore income levels) will build a certain amount of 'slack' into their budgets to allow for possible overspending. Central finance departments often impose maximum increases in spending or target levels to reduce the amount of slack in operational budgets.

Where management structures and responsibilities are not clearly defined and functional units are not all working in a coordinated manner towards the organization's overall strategic plan, individual units may try to maximize their own objectives at the expense of the organization's goals. This is referred to as *sub-optimality*.

A further concern is that in many health care systems much of the budget relates to clinical support – radiology, pathology and shared services such as administration, catering and laundry – rather than to direct costs (in the British NHS less than 50 per cent of the total budget of a clinical directorate relates to direct costs). Budget managers rarely have much influence over the allocation and apportionment (discussed in Chapter 4) of indirect costs and overheads although they make up a large part of their budgets. Managers should not be held responsible for those costs over which they have no control.

Finally, the analysis of budget variances, as described later in this chapter, may be seen as a way of apportioning blame for overspending or underperformance and this may be particularly demotivating for budget managers.

 Activity 7.3

> To what extent do you participate in your organization's budget-setting? How does your organization ensure that the highest possible standards are achieved and that there is no slack in the budget?

 Feedback

> Your answers to this question will reflect budgeting practice in your organization. In all organizations it is essential that those who are to be held responsible for a budget are actively involved in setting that budget. Unfortunately, this is not always what happens. While it is a good idea to organize a broad participation of staff, the problem is finding a balance between the demands for more resources and the economic constraints of the organization. This is reflected in the relationship between middle managers and top managers of an organization. In most organizations budget planning is a combination of a top-down and a bottom-up approach. Managers have a degree of freedom in contributing their own views to the budget but then have to adjust to meet the requirements of top management. A better way of reconciling both views is to agree and set targets for budget planning, for example:
>
> - administrative staff costs not to exceed 6 per cent of total staff costs
> - staff costs not to exceed inflation rates
>
> To make this work, middle managers need to be involved in the planning cycle in a way that enables participation at key decision points.

Approaches to budgeting

There are different ways in which budget-setting can be approached. Traditionally, the two most commonly encountered approaches were *incremental budgeting* and *zero-based budgeting*. In this section you will also learn about techniques which enable you to make your budget more accurate – *flexing*, which you have already come across in Chapter 3, and *profiling*.

Incremental budgeting

Incremental budgeting is the most commonly used approach to budgeting in both public and private sectors. It involves taking the previous year's budget as the starting point and concentrating on adjusting the figures to reflect the changes in planned activity levels and in costs and prices between the two years. This involves taking into account any change in planned activity as well as the level of inflation and projected pay rises.

Activity 7.4

This activity will give you practical experience in developing an incremental budget. The starting point is the 2005 budget based on the 'production' of 30,000 bed days, as shown in column 2 of Table 7.2.

Table 7.2 Incremental budget – working schedule

Budget heading	2005 budget (US$)	Additional activity in 2006 (US$)	Percentage increase in costs	Increase in costs due to pay rises/ inflation (US$)	2006 budget (US$)
Nursing pay	3 000 000	500 000	3	105 000	3 605 000
Non-pay costs	100 000				
Medical pay	760 000				
Management pay	300 000				
Consumables	340 000				
Admin pay	196 000				
Total	4 696 000				

In the year 2006:

- bed days planned are 35,000
- nursing and medical pay are expected to rise by 3 per cent
- management and administration pay are not expected to rise
- all other costs are expected to rise by 5 per cent

For the purposes of this activity assume that management costs are fixed but that all other costs are variable. Assume also that all pay rises take effect on 1 January 2006. Calculate the increases in activity and in cost levels to arrive at the budget for the year 2006. The first row of Table 7.2 has been filled in for you.

Feedback

Your completed schedule showing the incremental budget for 2006 should be as shown in Table 7.3.

Table 7.3 Incremental budget for 2006

Budget heading	2005 budget (US$)	Additional activity in 2006 (US$)	Percentage increase in costs	Increase in costs due to pay rises/ inflation (US$)	2006 budget (US$)
Nursing pay	3 000 000	500 000	3	105 000	3 605 000
Non-pay costs	100 000	16 667	5	3 500	120 167
Medical pay	760 000	126 667	3	26 600	913 267
Management pay	300 000	Nil	No increase	Nil	300 000
Consumables	340 000	56 667	5	19 833	416 500
Admin pay	196 000	32 667	No increase	Nil	228 667
Total	4 696 000	732 668	–	154 933	5 583 601

Zero-based budgeting

Zero-based budgeting, by contrast, assumes the previous year's budget to be quite irrelevant and begins from scratch to identify and cost all of the inputs that will be required to achieve the desired level of activity. Such an approach requires a radical reappraisal of the way in which resources are allocated. It challenges historical patterns of resource use and requires an awareness of needs and priorities as well as a detailed knowledge of the processes and jobs involved. This all makes zero-based budgeting a time-consuming and expensive exercise. However, it is worthwhile considering for discrete spending items or processes for which there are alternatives available, and for new programmes and projects.

Activity-based or flexible budgeting

Both incremental and zero-based budgets take the level of activity for the budget year as fixed. Increasingly, however, health services managers are adopting *flexible budgeting* systems designed to respond to changes in activity as the budget period progresses. This involves using cost information to calculate standard costs for the various items in a budget, so that the increase or decrease in expenditure associated with an activity level different from that which was budgeted can be forecast. Standard costs are usually based on historical cost information and should be regularly updated to reflect current costs.

You saw in Chapter 3 how flexible budgets can be constructed based on an understanding of costs and how they behave. The following activity requires you to construct a flexible budget for a radiology department.

 Activity 7.5

A radiology department expects to undertake 100 000 investigations for the year 2006 and plans to employ the resources shown in column one of Table 7.4.

Table 7.4 Budget for a radiology department

Budget heading	Base budget (100 000 investigations) (US$)	Budget per unit (standard cost) (US$)	Budget for additional activity (US$)	Adjusted (flexed) budget (US$)
X-ray film	250 000	2.500		
X-ray chemicals	43 200	0.432		
Radiopharmaceuticals	44 600	0.446		
Radiological protection	8 000	0.080		
Disposables	3 000	0.030		
Total	348 800	3.488		

After month three, it becomes clear that the department is more likely to undertake 110,000 investigations over the year. Adjust the budget to reflect this.

Feedback

Check your flexed budget against that shown below.

Table 7.5 Budget for a radiology department

Budget heading	Base budget (100 000 investigations) (US$)	Budget per unit (standard cost) (US$)	Budget for additional activity (US$)	Adjusted (flexed) budget (US$)
X-ray film	250 000	2.500	25 000	275 000
X-ray chemicals	43 200	0.432	4 320	47 520
Radiopharmaceuticals	44 600	0.446	4 460	49 060
Radiological protection	8 000	0.080	800	8 800
Disposables	3 000	0.030	300	3 300
Total	348 800	3.488	34 880	383 680

A fixed budget would not recognize the resource consequences of the additional activity. Consequently, the budget report would reflect the increased consumption of resources as an overspend (an adverse variance).

Profiling

Up to this point you have looked only at examples of annual budgets. However, if budgets are to be used for monitoring and control purposes it is necessary to break the budget down into smaller periods – months, weeks or even days. One way of doing this would be to divide the annual budget figure under each heading by 12 if you intended to review budgets on a monthly basis, by 52 for budgets to be reviewed weekly and so on. However, in many health services there is a marked seasonal variation in the level of activity. In summer, for example, there is likely to be a fall in the demand for treating patients with infectious diseases so that the need for agency nurses is likely to fall and heating costs will also fall. *Profiling* is simply the technique used to adjust for such seasonal variations within a budget, so that actual progress can be monitored against the budget.

The profile of a budget for agency nurses, doctors and heating costs for the four quarters of a year, for example, is as shown in Table 7.6. While doctors' costs are expected to be incurred evenly over the course of the year, the costs of agency nursing and heating are profiled to be greater in the winter months. Profiling is also an essential feature of budgets that are to be used for cash planning purposes.

Table 7.6 Budget profile for agency nursing, consultants and heating

	Apr–Jun (US$)	Jul–Sep (US$)	Oct–Dec (US$)	Jan–Mar (US$)	Total (US$)
Agency nursing	35 000	15 000	15 000	35 000	100 000
Doctors	50 000	50 000	50 000	50 000	200 000
Heating	32 000	16 000	48 000	64 000	160 000
Total	117 000	81 000	113 000	149 000	460 000

Budgets and control

Once a budget has been agreed and implemented, the budget-holders should receive regular reports showing actual expenditure to date. These reports are designed in such a way as to enable the comparison of budgeted and actual figures. A *variance* arises when the actual result is different from the budgeted result. Variances may be favourable, for example, an expenditure item that is underspent, or adverse, for an overspend under an expenditure heading. Table 7.7 is a simplified example of an extract from a budget report for the period 1 April to 30 September using the profiles shown in Table 7.6. The budget is not flexed.

Table 7.7 Budget report for the period I April to 30 September

	Budgeted expenditure (US$)	Actual expenditure (US$)	Variance (US$(000))
Doctors	100 000	100 000	Nil
Agency nursing	50 000	40 000	10F*
Heating	48 000	40 000	8F*
Disposables	10 000	14 000	4(A)*

* F indicates a favourable variance, (A) indicates an adverse (negative) variance

In this example expenditure on doctors was as budgeted, while there were favourable variances on the expenditure on both agency nursing and heating. There was an adverse variance in the expenditure on disposables. The budget-holder should be able to explain the circumstances that contributed to this position. Milder weather throughout the period may have led to fewer admissions and to a lower expenditure on heating, but why should there be such a significant adverse variance in the expenditure on disposables?

A variance may occur because:

- you have used more or fewer resources than planned – this is referred to as a usage or volume variance or, in the case of labour or overhead costs, an efficiency variance;
- the cost of those resources was greater or lower than anticipated (a price variance).

Figure 7.2 summarizes the range of situations associated with variances occurring for different reasons.

Variance analysis

It is possible to analyse variances so as to identify their underlying cause. Analysing variances into volume and price components is a skill that will help you to manage your budget and use your resources effectively.

This can be a complex undertaking in health services and will usually be done by the accounting department in consultation with departmental managers, setting up standard costs against which variances can be analysed. The example given here is a simplified one.

A pathology laboratory has established the following monthly budget:

- staff costs $25,000
- non-staff costs $15,000

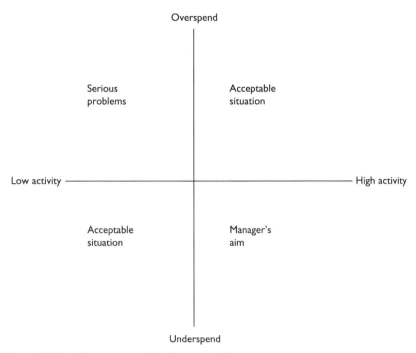

Figure 7.2 Possible outcomes of budgetary analysis

The planned activity level is 5000 tests each month. The monthly report provides the following information:

• 4500 tests were carried out
• staff costs $30,000
• non-staff costs $12,000

Clearly the number of appointments has not been met, yet staff costs have actually increased while non-staff costs are below the budgeted level. There may be several very obvious reasons for these variances, some of which (e.g. a pay award to certain grades of staff) are beyond the control of the manager. Nevertheless, by under-taking an analysis of the variances, the manager will get a clearer insight into the scale of the problems (see Table 7.8).

Table 7.8 Budget report for pathology laboratory

	Budget (US$)	Standard quantity tests	Standard costs per test (US$)	Actual costs (US$)	Actual quantity tests	Actual costs per test (US$)	Variance (US$)
Staff costs	25 000	5 000	5	30 000	4 500	6.666	5 000 (A)
Non-staff	15 000	5 000	3	12 000	4 500	2.666	3 000 F
Total	40 000			42 000			2 000 (A)

The formulae for calculating variances are as follows:

Cost variance = actual quantity × (standard cost – actual cost)

Efficiency variance = standard cost × (standard quantity – actual quantity)

Staff variances

The report shows an adverse variance of $5000 on staff expenditure. But there are two things to notice on the staff line of the report:

- The number of tests performed is 500 fewer than budgeted for.
- The actual cost per test is $6.67, whereas the budget, based on the standard cost, was $5.00 per test.

The variance of $5000 may be partly due to the fact that staff costs have increased, but what was the effect of the reduction in the number of tests performed?

Using the above formulae:

The cost variance is calculated as $4500 \times (5 - 6.666) = (\$7500)$

The efficiency variance is calculated as $5.00 \times (5000 - 4500) = \$2500$

The (adverse) cost variance is $7500, but the effect of this is actually offset or lessened by a favourable efficiency variance of $2500, giving a net variance of $5000. Note that the efficiency variance is based on the standard cost of $5 per unit and calculates the notional cost saving due to efficiency had the standard cost remained the same.

Non-staff variances

The report shows a favourable variance on non-staff expenditure of $3000. The actual cost per unit for non-staff items is only 33 cents lower than the standard cost. This indicates that the variance is likely to be in part attributable to an increase in efficiency as well as to a reduction in cost.

 Activity 7.6

Use the formulae for analysing variances to calculate the cost and efficiency variances on non-staff expenditure in the pathology department.

 Feedback

You should have analysed the variances as follows:

- cost variance = $4500 \times (3 - 2.666) = \$1500$
- efficiency variance = $3 \times (5000 - 4500) = \$1500$

As suggested above the favourable variance is partly due to a reduction in the cost and partly due to an increase in efficiency. The two variances when added together give a total of $3000 which is the figure shown in the report.

The manager should analyse the reasons for these variances carefully: the supplies variance is hugely favourable; would it be possible that cheap supplies are causing extra work for the laboratory staff? It is not possible to confirm all this without further investigation, but it does indicate what questions you might ask about performance and to whom you might talk about it.

Activity 7.7

Write down what you see as the benefits of variance analysis as described here.

Feedback

You might have noted that it is very helpful to analyse activities and find out the reasons why budgeted performance is different from actual performance. This helps establish a shared understanding between all those involved in service delivery as to what is happening and what needs to be done to improve performance. The alternative, where no one is sure of what is going on, can only lead to conflict which can never be resolved, and perceptions of unfairness by those on the losing side. It is important, though, to recognize that there is a danger that budget reports and variance analysis will be seen as tools for allocating blame. This can have severe demotivational effects on budget-holders.

Applying variance analysis to your own unit

Variance analysis applies to any unit that has a budget, including your own. Note, however, that you may encounter different terminology – for example, efficiency variances may be refered to as volume or usage variances and cost variances may be referred to as price variances. Activity 7.8 allows you to apply what you have learned in analysing your unit's budget report. Clearly it will not be relevant if your unit does not have its own budget but you are strongly encouraged to carry out the exercise if you can access the necessary figures.

Activity 7.8

As the final stage for this important skill you are asked to analyse the variances for two cost items in your own unit. For this it is suggested you pick two cost items and calculate the usage and cost variances for each item. This will give you experience of applying this technique in your work setting and demonstrate in a very practical and valuable way that you have mastered the material in this chapter. Complete your variance analysis using the table below.

Table 7.9 Variance analysis schedule (to be completed)

Cost category	Calculation	Variance	Adverse or favourable?
Cost variance			
Usage variance			
Cost variance			
Usage variance			

Feedback

Were you able to separate out cost and usage variances? This exercise demonstrates the importance of having access to all the necessary information in order to analyse variances.

Budgeting approaches reviewed

In this chapter you have seen several different approaches to budgeting. Incremental and zero-based budgeting are methods for constructing cost budgets. Once the budgets have been approved, one approach may be for them to remain fixed for the duration of the budget period. Fixed budgets have become a central tool in health services, enabling managers to implement the central strategy and contain costs. Flexible budgeting techniques using standard costing methods allow budget managers to review and analyse performance in a fast-changing environment, when activity levels are likely to vary from those on which the budget was based. However, flexible budgets are less frequently used and they usually have an overall cap – which means they are flexible within the limits of agreed activity.

 Activity 7.9

List at least two advantages and one disadvantage or difficulty for:

1   Incremental budgeting.
2   Zero-based budgeting.
3   Flexible budgeting.

 Feedback

Table 7.10 shows some of the advantages and disadvantages you may have listed.

Table 7.10 Advantages and disadvantages of different approaches to budgeting

	Incremental budgeting	Zero-based budgeting	Flexible budgeting
Advantages	Simple to understand Simple to calculate Does not take a lot of time Can also be used when income increases at a marginal rate	Provides a realistic budget Addresses historical inefficiencies Updates the relationship between inputs and outputs Organizations establish realistic financial and operational goals	Links activity and financial resources Makes budgets realistic Budgets are responsive to activity levels Should reduce variances from the budget Increases accountability of resource consumers

| Disadvantages | Assumes the budget for the previous year was correct and that simply adding to the previous year's budget is sufficient
Builds on and magnifies existing mistakes | Time-consuming
Expensive
Resistance to change
historic funding patterns | May not take account of stepped increases in costs
Requires additional provisions to contain overall costs
Only useful where costs will be recovered at standard prices/tariffs (i.e. not for block contracts) |

Even if an incremental budgeting approach is used, managers will need to carry out a zero-based budgeting exercise every few years in order to ensure that changing resource requirements, brought about by changes in technology, are reflected in the budget. Where standard costs are used for flexible budgeting it is important to ensure that they are up to date.

Summary

In this chapter you have learned how budgets are a management accountancy tool used to plan the consumption of resources over time. Budgets are set at every level within health systems including national, regional, organizational and departmental levels. The main purpose of budgeting is to control organizational activity by providing information for planning, performance measurement and measuring accountability. There are two main approaches to budgeting – incremental and zero-based. Activity-based or flexible budgeting allows budget-holders to adjust their budgets to reflect changes from the planned level of activity. Budgets are profiled over the budget period to take into account seasonal fluctuations in resource use. Variance analysis enables you to distinguish between cost variances and efficiency variances to enable effective budgetary control.

In the next chapter you will learn about the budget-setting process in health services.

References

Cook, A. (1995) Management accounting, in J. Simpson and R. Smith (eds) *Management for Doctors*. London: BMJ Publishing.

Drury, C. (1996) *Management and Cost Accounting*, 4th edn. London: International Thomson Business Press.

Garbutt, D. (1992) *Making Budgets Work*. London: Chartered Institute of Management Accountants.

Mellett, H., Marriott, N. and Harries, S. (1993) *Financial Management in the NHS: A Manager's Handbook*. London: Chapman & Hall.

8 The budgeting process

Overview

In the last chapter much of the emphasis was on how to use budget techniques when costing and analysing resource budgets for departments. But these budgets form part of a broader picture; there is a range of different types of budget which you need to know about when talking with financial experts. In this chapter you will examine the bigger strategic overview on budgets and how this is reflected in decisions concerning service developments. When you have completed this chapter you will have this overview and some sharp insights into management decision-making on service developments.

Learning objectives

By the end of this chapter you should be able to:

- **describe different types of budget and explain their purposes**
- **describe different approaches to preparing budgets**
- **identify how budgetary approaches fit into the bigger picture of an overall budget strategy**
- **evaluate the impact on a balanced budget strategy of decisions to outsource services**

Key terms

Balanced budget strategy A strategy that ensures that the total of all expenditure budgets is equal to the total income budget.

Capital budgets Budgets that relate to items appearing in the balance sheet, such as the acquisition or disposal of property belonging to the organization.

Cash budgets (cash flow forecasts) Budgets which profile cash flows over the budget period, to ensure that there is enough cash to meet operational and other needs.

Master budget The coordinated overall budget which combines the functional budgets, the capital budget and the cash flow budget with the budgeted income statement and balance sheet for the forthcoming period.

Revenue budgets Budgets that relate to items in the operational activities of the organization.

Staff budgets Budgets that detail staff numbers at all levels and associated staff costs.

Budgets in context

There are many different types of budget covering all aspects of the organization's operations. Broadly, there are two main categories of budget:

- *revenue budgets* that relate to items appearing in the income statement, that is items relating to the operational activities of the organization;
- *capital budgets* that relate to items appearing in the balance sheet, such as the acquisition or disposal of property belonging to the organization.

You will remember that these statements were introduced in Chapter 2, and you will be returning to them in Chapters 9 to 14.

Cash budgets, which profile cash flows over the budget period, ensure that there is enough cash to meet operational and other needs. All of the budgets within an organization will be combined by its financial managers to form a *master budget*. This may be translated into a forecast income statement and a forecast balance sheet showing the organization's planned position at the end of the budget period.

The budgeting process is normally closely prescribed by the finance department. The various cost centre managers are advised as to the contracted activity levels for the forthcoming year and are required to calculate the expected costs to their department of carrying out these activities. These resource budgets are then reviewed and collated by the finance department with other budgets to form the master budget.

The two main budgets for most clinical departments will be staff budgets and non-staff budgets. Other budgets used include cross charges budgets, capital charges budgets (described below), capital budgets and income budgets. However, in your own organization these may be called by different names.

Staff budgets

Staff costs are the biggest cost item of all in many health care organizations. It requires careful and thorough planning to ensure the service is staffed at the right level. Once you have the agreed activity level for the forthcoming year, the first step in constructing a staff budget is to identify and list the number of posts and their associated costs. (The finance department will provide details of payscales and of staff-related costs such as pension contributions and staff benefits.) The numbers and grades of staff employed are generally prescribed through some system of human resource control. Within case-mix systems the number of projected cases can be used to determine the required staffing levels for the agreed contracts; in more traditional systems an incremental approach might be used, with last year's staffing levels being adjusted to reflect any planned change in activity levels. Where staff are employed in more than one department, or part-time or contract staff are employed, their cost is calculated as a fraction of a full-time post (referred to as a full-time equivalent). Where a staff member works in more than one department, systems should be in place to ensure that their full costs are allocated between different departments – the organization's staff budgets, when added up, should equal total staff costs.

There are several things that must be considered when drawing up a staff budget:

- Will staffing levels change during the year? If so, the budget profile should show when these changes will take place and reflect the resulting changes in staff costs.
- Are there any pending or anticipated pay rises? If so, what grades of staff will be entitled to pay increases, what will be the level of these increases and when will they come into effect?
- If you have surplus staff it is costing you money that could be used elsewhere where it is really needed. However, you need to allow for staff vacancies, training and holidays.
- What is the likelihood that the planned activity level will vary and what flexibility do you have to respond immediately to this variation? If there is flexible support available from other departments in time of need then you will have very good reason to minimize your staffing. If this is not the case then you probably need to be more cautious.

Staff budgets are a vital part of the overall budget. Activity 8.1 is intended to give you the opportunity to discover for yourself how staff budgets are constructed in your own organization.

 Activity 8.1

1 List the steps taken and explain how to plan and budget for staff costs in your department or another department in your organization with which you are familiar.
2 Your investigation into how you plan and budget for staff costs will have highlighted aspects of the planning and budgeting process that could be improved. So, explain here how you consider this process could be improved, indicating any priorities you have.

 Feedback

1 Your review of planning and budgeting for staff should include reference to:

- activity
- measuring staff productivity
- forecasting of workload
- variability in workload
- staff grades and whole time equivalents (WTEs)
- staff vacancies
- training
- holidays
- sickness
- flexible support available from outside the department
- emergency cover arrangements
- pay rises

- pay/grade drift
- skill mix changes.

2 You may wish to discuss any concerns you have identified with colleagues either in your own department or in the finance department.

Non-staff budgets

As in Chapter 7, non-staff costs are referred to here under a single heading, although this heading covers a diverse range of costs from drugs and medical supplies to heating and electricity. The starting point, as with staff budgets, is the level of activity (patient volume and case mix) for the forthcoming year. The approach to this will depend on whether the organization uses a case-mix system that allows for DRG budgeting, in which case a zero-based approach can be used based on the projected numbers of cases. More traditionally, an incremental approach is adopted, with adjustments being made to the previous year's budget to reflect planned changes in activity levels.

Other questions which should be asked are as follows:

- Are there any 'one-off' or non-recurring items that should be included?
- What is the likely effect of any anticipated price rises? In some health services, departmental budgets will automatically be increased to reflect price changes as they occur.
- How would changes in the planned level of activity affect the various items in this budget?

Many of the costs may not be spread evenly over the budget period, so the next step will be to profile the expenditure over the 12-month budget period (usually on a monthly basis), as discussed in Chapter 7.

Where there are significant changes either in resource use or in prices during the year the non-staff budget will need to be adjusted and updated to reflect these changes.

Cross charges

The practice of cross-charging or recharging the cost of work done by one department for another is common to many organizations. So, for example, the costs of radiology, laundry and catering provided to an orthopaedic ward should all be included in the budget for that ward. It is sometimes argued that the support departments have little incentive to control their costs if they merely pass them all on. However, standard costing systems as described in Chapter 7 provide the information necessary to budget for cross charges on the basis of activity levels and provide an incentive for support departments to contain their costs.

Capital charges

In addition to the staff and non-staff costs, organizations also have to budget for the replacement and renewal of equipment and facilities. Capital charges are a notional charge relating to the use of capital equipment or of land and buildings which have been purchased and which may need replacing in the future. Capital charges include depreciation, the charge to expenditure over the lifetime of the asset. Responsibility for capital charges budgets will be given to those who will control the purchasing decisions concerning the use and replacement of equipment. While departmental budgets are likely to include capital charges in respect of equipment they are less likely to include capital charges in respect of land and buildings.

Capital budgets

As you saw at the beginning of Chapter 7, senior managers must engage in longer-term strategic planning. Organizations will need to have plans for the updating and eventual replacement of existing facilities as well as for their expansion to accommodate increased levels of activity. The costs associated with these plans will feed into the capital budgets that form part of the annual budget.

Income budgets

Up to this point the focus has been on costs. It is vital that the organization can be sure that it has secured the necessary income to fund the resource use associated with the planned level of activity. An income budget is produced to show the planned levels of activity and the associated sources of income over the budget period. The responsibility for the income budget will normally lie within the finance department.

When negotiating contracts, health services providers may include a provision for inflation. This provision may be held in a separate 'reserve' account until such time as price increases actually take effect and departmental budgets are adjusted accordingly.

The cash budget

One of the main functions of the finance department is to ensure that cash due to the organization is received promptly and that there is enough money in the bank to pay staff salaries and suppliers. To do this, the finance department will collate all of the profiled budgets to produce a profiled cash budget for the period. This will include all expenditure and revenue that will give rise to cash flows but will exclude 'non-cash' expenditure items such as notional capital charges. Once the information from the budgets is collated it may be necessary to go back and make adjustment to some of the subsidiary budgets to ensure that the cash flow is balanced at all times. The cash budget is the most vital of all and it is reviewed on a regular basis.

Balanced budget strategy

Budgets need to be balanced: that means there have to be ways to ensure that the appropriate balance between income and expenditure is maintained so that the organization can pay its way. When potential service developments are considered, their impact should be evaluated against the need to keep the budget balanced.

The fundamental rule is that for whatever costs are planned there must be the equivalent amount of planned income. That sounds like good sense but it is surprisingly easy to overlook either by wishful thinking or the assumption that somehow things will muddle through as they did last year.

Health services cannot make detailed plans for expenditure unless they have secured a funding source for the provision of services that will result in that expenditure. This is referred to as a *balanced budget strategy*, that is, the total of all expenditure budgets should be equal to the total income budget; it is a fundamental requirement in any organization. To achieve a balanced budget strategy, all types of income must be identified – for example, payments from financial intermediaries as well as co-payments and user fees. Where contracts are used to pay providers, these need to identify the planned level of activity and the total price to be charged for that activity, and state clearly the adjustments to be made if activity levels are higher or lower than planned.

In practice, budgets are often balanced by the inclusion of non-recurrent or one-off funding solutions. It is important to recognize that short-term strategies of this kind can lead to underlying recurrent financial difficulties. Where such situations do arise, there should be a plan in place to ensure that the organization recovers from the imbalance.

Contract changes during the budget period

Any changes in income from those in the original income budget must be reflected in budget reports generated during the year. There are, however, different ways of dealing with them.

Consider the case where a hospital's contract is altered to include a further 200 day surgery cases generating a further $10,000 in income, but generating a further $10,000 in expenditure in the day surgery department. One way would simply be to reflect the additional $10,000 as a favourable variance in the income budget and as an adverse variance of $10,000 in the day surgery budget. These variances would cancel each other out, but it would not be clear from the budget report that the increase in expenditure was actually due to an increase in activity. An alternative solution would be to produce updated budgets reflecting the increased number of day cases and the increased costs resulting from them. The increased income would be balanced by the increased costs. This is a simplistic example because it does not take into account any contribution to fixed costs that the additional contract might make, but it does illustrate the balanced budget approach.

Getting to know your budget system

As a manager you need to be able to navigate your way around the budget system in your own organization so that you understand where and how all the bits of the budget jigsaw fit together. Completing the next activity will help you do this.

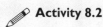 **Activity 8.2**

Listed in Table 8.1 are some budgets often used in health service organizations that will probably have equivalents in your own organization. You need to identify what the equivalent budget is for your organization and give examples of the main items that are in it to complete the table.

Depending on the size of your organization, you should be able to identify several other budgets in addition to the ones already listed. These should fit together into your own comprehensive picture of your budget system, which includes both income and expenditure, capital spending and fixed assets, and cash flow.

In addition identify any budgets not listed in Table 8.1.

Table 8.1 Some budgets used in health service organizations

Budget type	Equivalent name for this budget in your organization	Examples of the main items included in your budget
Income budgets		
Staff budgets		
Non-staff budgets		
Capital charges budgets		
Recharges budgets		

Deciding whether to buy in services

A major decision that affects all organizations is making choices on what services to provide in-house and what services to buy in from outside. If the service is cheaper and better from outside, the decision is clear: cease providing the service in-house and award a contract for the service to an outside provider. But, and it is a huge but, can anyone be certain it is cheaper? By carefully analysing the costs and costing the service as it is provided in-house, a decision can be made. Normally for the purpose of contracting-out, a market testing exercise is performed, inviting providers from outside the organization to bid for a tender. Contracting-out is only suitable for functions and services that can easily be separated from the organization's core services, such as cleaning, catering or laundry or medical support services. For the tender document a careful specification of the desired quantity and quality of the service is required. When the bids are evaluated the organization should only go ahead with the project if the expected efficiency gains materialize in an acceptable period of time and are sustainable in the long run.

✎ Activity 8.3

This activity deals with just this kind of decision: whether to do something in-house or not. As the following summary shows, it can be difficult to realize the benefits of outsourcing if the organization is not able to reduce fixed costs.

The Windward Hospital has a laundry department which provides services for all hospital wards. However, recently a newly-launched commercial laundry service has approached several budget managers with a view to providing a cost-effective alternative of equal quality to the service provided by the hospital.

Costs for the hospital's laundry department for 2004 are shown in Table 8.2.

Table 8.2 Windward Hospital laundry department costs for 2004

	$(000)
Direct costs:	
Staff costs	50
Consumables	5
Overheads and cross charges inward:	
Capital charges	3
Energy	10
Housekeeping	10
Maintenance	5
Administration	10
Total costs	93

During the year the laundry processed 150,000 items of linen, 18,000 of which were charged to the surgical ward on a standard cost basis. (For simplicity it is assumed that all items of linen have the same standard cost.) The budgets for the forthcoming year have already been set on the basis that there will be no change in the laundry budget over the previous year and that there will be no change in the surgical ward's laundry services requirements.

The manager of a surgical ward thinks that buying in laundry services may save money. The commercial laundry quotes $50 per 100 items for 18,000 items over a one-year period.

1   First, calculate the standard cost per item of linen, using Table 8.3 below. The calculation of standard costs is a matter of dividing each cost by the planned activity. This is also the rate used for recharges.
2   Think very carefully about the implications, both for the ward manager's budget and for the hospital as a whole, of deciding to buy in the laundry service. Write a memo (in point form) from the finance department to the manager of the surgical ward explaining the true cost of using the services of the commercial laundry.

Table 8.3 Standard cost calculations for the Windward Hospital laundry

	Cost $(000)	Items (000)	Standard cost $
Staff			
Consumables			
Overheads and cross charges			
Totals			

Feedback

1   Compare your standard cost calculations with those in Table 8.4.

Table 8.4 Standard costs for the Windward Hospital laundry

	Cost $(000)	Items (000)	Standard cost $
Staff	50	150	0.33
Consumables	5	150	0.03
Overheads and cross charges	38	150	0.25
Totals	93	150	0.61

2   Your memo to the surgical ward manager should have included the following points:

- Standard costs for the in-house laundry service are 0.61 per item.
- For 18,000 items this would be a cost to the surgical ward for the forthcoming year of $10,980.
- Buying in the laundry service would cost $50 per 100 items, making a total cost of $9000 for the year.
- The saving to the surgical ward would be $1980.
- The cross charge income of the in-house laundry would be reduced by $10,980.
- In the short term the direct costs of the laundry would only be reduced by the cost of the consumables associated with the laundry service provided for the surgical ward (0.03 × 18,000, or $540), because it will not be possible to make an immediate reduction in the staffing levels, cross charges or overheads.
- The laundry's budget would result in an adverse variance of $10,980 under cross charges and a favourable variance of $540 under consumables.

- The only way that the laundry could make this up would be by increasing its cross charges to other departments (which is unlikely to happen once budgets have been agreed).
- Although there is an apparent saving of $1980 to the surgical ward, the actual cost to the hospital if the surgical ward were to buy in laundry services would be $10,440, although this may be reduced in the longer term, if the laundry makes staff reductions and reduces its overhead costs as a result of the decrease in workload.

The main thing you need to recognize is that only the variable costs will be saved if the laundry service is bought in. The fixed costs will still be incurred. This is the overheads trap: overheads can look like variable costs when expressed as a standard cost per unit but overall these overheads are really fixed costs. So in this example it will cost more to buy in the service than to do it internally in the first place. This shows that when a service development in a specific area is proposed, its effects on the entire organization need to be carefully considered. For central management this has the implication that unit managers should not be given discretion to decide on outsourcing in areas that affect other units or the organization as a whole.

Summary

In this chapter you have seen how every organization will prepare a range of budgets covering every aspect of its activity. These will include manpower or staff budgets, other resource budgets, income budgets, capital budgets, cash budgets and a master budget reflecting the overall impact of all of these on the organization. The fundamental resource planning rule is that planned income should meet expenditure, that is, a balanced budget strategy should be maintained. Staff budgets form the major part of most expenditure budgets in health services. They should be drawn up with reference to activity and workload forecasting, productivity, staff numbers, grades and vacancies, training, sickness, holidays, outside support and emergency cover, as well as to pay scales. When using standard costs to decide whether to buy in services from outside it is important not to lose sight of the fact that the fixed costs included in the standard cost calculation will continue to be incurred in the short run.

SECTION 3

Financial accounting

9 | Introduction to financial accounting

Overview

This is the first of six chapters concerned with financial accounting. Financial accounting is the process whereby an organization keeps a detailed record of all of its business transactions, enabling it to ensure that payments are made on time and that the organization receives the payments that are due to it. The accounting records are also used to produce statements summarizing the organization's financial performance. Chapters 9–14 are concerned with financial accounting; this chapter begins with an overview of financial accounting, the purposes it serves, the concepts on which it is based and the way in which it is regulated. You will then go on in subsequent chapters to learn about the financial statements – the income statement, the balance sheet and the cash flow statement – and to get some practical experience of analysing and interpreting these statements.

Learning objectives

By the end of this chapter you should be able to:

- **identify the users of financial accounts**
- **explain why it is necessary to produce financial statements**
- **define double entry bookkeeping**
- **discuss the concepts on which financial accounting is based**

Key terms

Accruals accounting An accounting system that recognizes revenue or costs as earned in the period when the transaction takes place (in contrast to cash accounting which only records transactions when cash is received or paid).

Asset Something that is owned by the organization; assets represent the *use* of organizational funds.

Balance sheet A statement of the total assets, liabilities and capital of an organization at a given moment.

Capital The funds invested in the organization by its owner or owners (accountancy definition).

Cash flow statement A statement summarizing the inflows and outflows of cash over the accounting period.

Double entry book-keeping A system of record-keeping which recognizes that there are two sides to every transaction.

Entity concept The unit for which the accounts are prepared; separate and distinct from its employees.

Going concern Assumes the entity will continue to exist into the foreseeable future, and there is no intention to close it down or make drastic operational cutbacks.

Historic and current costs Historic cost reflects the original cost of an asset, current cost reflects the replacement cost.

Income statement (income and expenditure account) A summary of income and expenditure over a period of time.

Liability Something that is owed by the organization; liabilities represent the *source* of funds.

Materiality Those items that are significant enough to affect evaluation or decisions.

Money measurement Those items to which a monetary value can be attributed included in the accounts.

Prudence (conservatism) A concept that requires all costs or losses to be recognized as soon as they are foreseen, not to record anticipated profits until actually realized.

Stakeholders An individual or group with a substantive interest in an issue (ie interest group), including those with some role in making a decision or its execution.

Trial balance A list of all the balances in an organization's book of account; this is usually the first step in preparing the annual accounts.

To whom is a health care organization responsible?

As in large business organizations, very few health care organizations are run by the people who own them. Owners include:

- the state;
- national or international agencies;
- charitable trusts or foundations;
- medical insurance companies;
- institutional investors such as large pension companies;
- private investors.

The people who manage organizations are therefore held accountable to the owners for stewardship of the funds (capital) with which they have been entrusted. In addition, organizations may have many other interested parties or *stakeholders* who wish to reassure themselves that the organization is being managed in their best interests. The chief executive of a health care organization may be accountable to:

- a board of directors of the organization;
- a public health authority;
- patients;
- charities and other sponsors;
- medical insurance companies;

- taxpayers;
- the medical and other professions;
- the employees of the organization.

How many of the above would you identify as stakeholders of the organization for which you work? Can you think of others that you would add to the list?

Organizations produce annual accounts designed to show their stakeholders how the resources entrusted to them have been used. In most countries legislation has been enacted to ensure that such accounts give a true and fair view of the organization's performance and financial standing. Such legislation requires that the financial statements be prepared according to certain concepts and principles, which will be discussed later in this chapter, and that their layout follows a specified format.

The need for a financial accounting system

As in all organizations, health care organizations have expenses to meet – salaries to be paid, drugs and other bills to be paid – they also have income payable to them from various sources. Accounting systems, whether they are manual (entered by hand in books of account) or computerized, help organizations to ensure that these transactions are conducted accurately and at the right time. They also provide a comprehensive record of the financial transactions that the organization has conducted. These records are used to compile the income and expenditure figures used in budget variance analysis as discussed in Chapter 7. At periodic intervals (usually annually) the records are summarized to produce accounts which will be available to stakeholders. Accounting periods are often selected by organizations to coincide with the fiscal (tax) year. In some countries the accounting period is the calendar year, in others organizations are free to specify their accounting period when the organization is registered.

The double entry book-keeping system

The basis of all financial accounting systems is *double entry book-keeping*, a system of record keeping first developed by an Italian merchant in the fifteenth century, which recognizes that there are two sides to every transaction. If, for example, you buy something for cash, then the effect of the transaction in your books of account will be to increase your stock of assets (the item you bought), while at the same time reducing the amount of cash you hold. Each transaction involves two entries, referred to as debit and credit entries.

Double entry book-keeping reflects that each financial transaction has a *giver* and a *receiver*, in other words it describes the 'sources' and 'uses' of funds. Understanding the terminology used in financial accounting is what non-accountants find most challenging. However, it is quite simple once you have understood the basic principle of double entry book-keeping.

- An *asset* is something that will be used in running the organization; it represents the *use* of organizational funds.
- A *liability* refers to how the asset is funded – the *source* of funds.
- Another source of funds is *capital* – the funds invested in the organization by its owner or owners. (The organization is regarded for accounting purposes as an

entity with a separate identity from its owners.) You should note, however, that in Chapters 1 and 2 'capital' was used in the economic sense to refer to physical assets (such as land, buildings and equipment).

Thus if you buy a car on credit:

- you have an asset – the car;
- you have a liability – the finance company.

If you bought the car using cash, you would have:

- an additional asset – the car;
- less of another asset – cash.

All assets of an organization are at any time equal to its owners' capital plus any outstanding liabilities. This identity is referred to as 'the accounting equation':

Assets = capital + liabilities

A basic understanding of how the various forms of transactions affect the balance between assets and liabilities in the double entry system will help you understand the more complex financial accounts you are going to consider in this and the following chapters. Activity 9.1 is designed to give you this basic understanding.

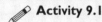 **Activity 9.1**

Assume you have received a starting capital of $20,000 in cash from government to open a new health centre. As you will have to use $14,000 to pay staff, the remaining $6000 won't allow you to buy both a vehicle and the equipment which is required for the operation of the facility. An opening statement for the health centre would look as in Table 9.1.

Table 9.1 New health centre – opening statement

Sources of funds	$	Uses of funds	$
Capital	20 000		
Liabilities		Assets	
	0	Cash	20 000
Total	20 000		20 000

Your first action is to spend $4000 of the cash on a vehicle. Purchasing the vehicle means that one asset (the vehicle) is created while the other (cash) decreases. Liabilities remain unchanged. The statement would be as in Table 9.2.

Table 9.2 Statement after buying one vehicle

Sources of funds		Uses of funds	
Capital	20 000		
Liabilities		Assets	
		Cash	16 000
		Vehicle	4 000
Total	20 000		20 000

In the first week you then carry out the following transactions. Show how the statement shown in Table 9.2 would change after each of the following three transactions:

1 Buy equipment worth $5000 on credit.
2 Use $2000 cash for a part repayment to equipment supplier.
3 Raise $2000 bank overdraft to make further payment to supplier.

Feedback

1 Buying equipment on credit will create a liability that is balanced by an asset of the same amount. Total assets and liabilities go up by $5000 (Table 9.3).

Table 9.3 Statement after buying medical equipment on credit

Sources of funds		Uses of funds	
Capital	20 000		
Liabilities		Assets	
Creditors	5 000	Cash	16 000
		Equipment	5 000
		Vehicle	4 000
Total	25 000		25 000

2 Using cash to pay a creditor reduces assets and liabilities by that amount (Table 9.4).

Table 9.4 Statement after part repayment

Sources of funds		Uses of funds	
Capital	20 000		
Liabilities		Assets	
Creditors	3 000	Cash	14 000
		Equipment	5 000
		Vehicle	4 000
Total	23 000		23 000

3 Raising a bank overdraft to make a further repayment to the creditor creates a new liability, but it reduces the existing liability to the equipment supplier by the same amount (Table 9.5).

Table 9.5 Statement after raising bank overdraft to pay creditor

Sources of funds		Uses of funds	
Capital	20 000		
Liabilities		Assets	
Creditors	1 000	Cash	14 000
Bank overdraft	2 000	Equipment	5 000
		Vehicle	4 000
Total	23 000		23 000

Of course you would not draw up a statement after each transaction in this way. You would merely enter the transactions into the accounting system when they occurred and they would be reflected in the periodic financial statements. However, the point of this activity was to illustrate the basic principle of the double entry system, that whatever the transaction, capital plus liabilities must equal total assets.

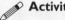 **Activity 9.2**

Complete the matrix in Table 9.6 on the effects of transactions in the double entry bookkeeping system. The effects of the first transaction have been entered for you.

Table 9.6 Effect of transactions in the double entry bookkeeping system

Transaction	Liabilities		Assets	
	Increase	Decrease	Increase	Decrease
Cash purchase			✓	✓
Credit purchase				
Cash payment to creditor				
Loan raised to pay creditor				

 Feedback

Compare your answers with Table 9.7.

Table 9.7 Effect of transactions in the double entry bookkeeping system (solution)

Transaction	Liabilities		Assets	
	Increase	Decrease	Increase	Decrease
Cash purchase			✓	✓
Credit purchase	✓		✓	
Cash payment to creditor		✓		✓
Loan raised to pay creditor	✓	✓		

Source: adapted from Buckley et al. (1997)

At the end of each accounting period the first test of accuracy is to ensure that the total debits is equal to the total credits. Thus a list of all balances, the *trial balance*, is prepared and it is this that forms the basis for the preparation of the financial statements.

The annual report and accounts

The annual report is usually drawn up to give full and detailed information on the organization and its activities over the previous accounting period. Increasingly, organizations use annual reports as an important way of informing their stake-holders about their mission and their organizational objectives, and the ways in which they are meeting them. To comply with statutory regulations, however, annual reports must also include written reviews by the chairman and the finance director, statements regarding the accounting principles and conventions used and a set of financial statements including:

- an income statement;
- a balance sheet;
- a cash flow statement.

These are summary statements and will be backed up with additional information to be found included in the notes to the accounts.

The income statement

The income statement summarizes income and expenditure over a period of time, usually a 12-month period in the case of statutory accounts. Note that you may be more familiar with the terms 'income and expenditure account' for a not-for-profit organization, or 'profit and loss account', but these will in due course be replaced by the International Accounting Committee's preferred 'income statement' (IASC 2004). The income statement for a health service organization will look something like the example shown in Table 9.8.

Table 9.8 Simplified example of an income statement for a health service

Income statement for the year ended 30 September 2004		
	$000	$000
Income:		
Contract income	68 545	
Private fees	12 345	80 890
Less operating expenses:		
Staff costs	60 345	
Supplies	14 555	
Depreciation	4 398	79 298
Operating surplus for the year		1 592
Interest payments	465	
Surplus (deficit) for the year		1 127

In practice these summaries will be supported by notes to the accounts providing further detail under each of the income and expenditure headings.

The balance sheet

In contrast to the income and expenditure statement which shows the transactions over a period of time, the balance sheet shows the assets, liabilities and capital of an organization as at a particular moment (on the last day of the accounting period). It is often described as a snapshot of the organization at a particular moment.

The statements in Tables 9.1 to 9.5 are balance sheets in their simplest form. In practice the standardized layout is rather different, as you will see as you work through Chapters 10 to 14.

It is important to note that the preparation of the income statement and balance sheet can only be undertaken after the end of the financial accounting period and it may take up to several months before the audited accounts are ready for publication. Thus they are historic statements and as such do not reflect the current state of affairs of the business.

Accruals accounting and the cash flow statement

The third financial accounting statement is designed to explain the cash flows to and from the organization during the accounting period in question. In order to understand the need for such a statement you need to know about *accruals accounting*.

The example of a new health centre, above, used accruals accounting: when an item was bought on credit, the statement of affairs reflected this as an increase in assets with a corresponding increase in the amount owing to creditors. This is an example of the accruals or matching concept, which states that transactions should be reflected in the organization's accounts in the period in which they take place. The alternative, which was historically favoured by many public sector organizations, is a cash accounting system, where transactions are only recorded when cash changes hands. Cash accounting is a simpler form of accounting and is still common in the health services of many low- and middle-income countries, though there is increasingly a move towards accruals accounting. Accruals accounting means that the income statement and the balance sheet together do not reflect the flow of funds into and out of the organization, as the following examples show:

- while income may have been entered into the accounting system because associated services have been carried out, the cash may still be owing to the organization, and will therefore be included in the debtors' accounts balance;
- the organization may have paid cash to creditors who were owed money in respect of transactions which took place in the previous accounting period.

An organization must be in a position to meet its obligations: it needs to have enough cash in the bank to meet its regular payroll commitments, pay its debts when they become due etc. In fact, cash is sometimes called the lifeblood of an organization. It is important that those responsible for financial management are able to show that the cash position of the organization is a healthy one.

To explain the flow of cash into and out of the organization during the accounting period, a *cash* or *funds flow statement* is included as one of the three main financial statements that an organization is required to produce and include in its annual report. This statement will be described in more detail in Chapter 12.

The role of external auditors

Most health care organizations, whether in the public or the private sector, are required by law to have their financial statements checked by independent auditors who are qualified to give an opinion on whether the accounts present a true and fair view of the state of affairs of the organization and comply with the accounting conventions as stated. The auditors will perform a thorough review of the accounting system, checking that procedures and controls are adequate for compiling the financial statements and ensuring compliance with accounting requirements. A qualified opinion will be given if the auditor is not satisfied that the accounts are materially correct.

Accounting principles

Accounting systems are designed to translate resource flows and organizational activity into financial terms. In order to do so, accountants follow certain concepts (or rules) and principles referred to as generally accepted accounting principles (GAAPs). In recent years there has been a move towards the development of Internationally Agreed Accounting Standards (IAS) and away from the system where each country had its own GAAP. This has been largely driven by the globalization of industry but a parallel set of standards, the International Public Sector Accounting Standards (IPSAS) has been agreed for public sector organizations. These are mostly based on the IAS.

While you do not need to know about the standards in detail, you should be aware of the following basic concepts:

1 The *entity concept* states that for accounting purposes the unit for which the accounts are prepared is quite separate and has a distinct existence from its employees.
2 The *going concern* concept assumes that the entity will continue to exist into the foreseeable future and that there is no intention to close it down or to make drastic operational cutbacks. This has implications for the value that is placed on assets that appear in the balance sheet, for if it were assumed that the entity would be closing down in the near future then assets could only be valued at their sale or scrap value. However, the going concern assumption allows accountants to spread the cost of an asset over its useful economic life.
3 The *money measurement* concept requires that only those items to which a monetary value can be attributed be included in the accounts. While assets which have been purchased have a clear monetary value, it is not so easy to put a value on the expertise of staff or the knowledge that may contribute to the organization's performance. In recent years commercial organizations have devised schemes to include these values on their balance sheets, for they argue that they significantly affect the value placed on the organization by investors. However, most health service organizations continue to observe the money measurement concept.
4 The *accruals* or matching concept, which you have already come across in the discussion of the need for a cash flow statement above, means that the accounts should include all transactions concluded during the accounting period and the cost of all resources consumed during that period. Under the accruals system

provision is made for items such as power consumed, even though a bill may not yet have been received.

5 The *consistency of presentation* concept states that in preparing accounts consistency should be observed by: treating similar items within a single set of accounts in the same way; using the same treatment for similar items between one accounting period and the next. This enables comparisons to be made between items and between the accounts for successive periods.

6 *Materiality* should be a consideration when deciding which financial facts should be included in the accounting statements and how they should be presented. While excessive detail should be avoided, summarization should not be taken too far.

7 The *prudence* (or *conservatism*) concept requires accountants to fully recognize all costs or losses as soon as they are foreseen but not to record an anticipated profit until it is actually realized. This concept is, however, subject to much debate. It can, for example, be seen as conflicting with the accruals concept and has mostly been replaced by the concept of fair presentation or a true and fair view.

In addition to the above, the IAS include a vast number of rules on the accounting treatment of asset values, depreciation, provisions and reserves, levels of disclosure and many other aspects of financial accounts. Many of these do not apply to health services and it is, in any case, the responsibility of the financial accountants within the organization to ensure they are observed. However, as you work through Chapters 10 and 11 you will come across the following accounting terms, which will be discussed in more detail:

• *depreciation:* the measure attached to the wearing out, using up or reduction in the useful economic life of tangible fixed assets such as machinery and equipment;

• *amortization:* the process of reducing or 'writing off' the value of an intangible fixed asset (such as a lease, a licence or research and development activities) over a period of time;

• *provisions:* amounts set aside out of the profits or surplus of an organization to cover a recognized liability; provisions for doubtful debts and for clinical negligence claims are examples;

• *reserves:* part of the capital of an organization, other than owners' capital; retained profits and revaluation reserves are examples.

An awareness of the concepts and terms outlined above will help you in your study of financial accounting.

Another important question is that of how to value transactions and assets for balance sheet purposes. The alternative approaches are *historic cost* valuation and *current cost* valuation. A commonly accepted approach is to value all 'revenue transactions' (purchase of supplies and other costs regularly incurred in running the organization) at their historic cost and to value capital transactions (purchase of assets including buildings and equipment) at their current or replacement cost. It is the responsibility of the directors to ensure that they include a statement of accounting policies in the financial statements, explaining their accounting treatment of assets and other items.

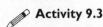 **Activity 9.3**

Now, as a quick test of your understanding of the various concepts, answer the following questions, in each case stating the concept on which you base your answer.

1 A hospital is awarded a large contract to provide health screening for a company's employees. Should it show the value of the contract in its books of account straight away?

2 A health centre has not yet paid its electricity bill for $500 when the accounts are being prepared. Should it be included?

3 A hospital has an internationally renowned team of neurosurgeons who attract many patients. How should their worth be reflected in the accounts?

4 A screening clinic has two scanners in constant use but the accountant is told they would have little or no scrap value. Should they be included in the accounts?

5 A new accountant thinks that an organization should change the way in which fixed assets are valued. What would you say?

 Feedback

1 No, the *conservatism* or *prudence* concept requires that income should not be anticipated before it is earned.

2 Yes, the *accruals* concept is relevant here; the financial impact of events should be entered into the accounts as the events occur, not when the related cash flow takes place.

3 There is no way of assigning a reasonably accurate monetary value to the team, so the *money measurement* concept states that their value should not be included in the accounts.

4 The *going concern* concept is relevant here; even though if the unit were to be closed down the scanners would have no value, they should be shown at their original or historic cost less the depreciation written off to date. They should continue to be listed in the schedule of fixed assets even though their value is zero.

5 *Consistency* requires that the same accounting treatment should be used between one period and the next. Where there is a valid reason for changing the accounting treatment, then this should be done with the approval of the auditors and the organization may be required to restate its results for previous accounting periods.

You will find that these principles are so fundamental that they have been enacted in the company laws of most countries as well as in the accounting standards.

Summary

Managers of health care organizations are accountable for the stewardship of funds entrusted to them. Financial accounting systems are designed to assist organizations to carry out and record all the organization's transactions. The double entry bookkeeping system is used to enter all transactions in the books of account and from these a list of balances known as a trial balance is produced. Summary financial statements produced on a regular basis keep stakeholders informed of the financial performance of the organization. These statements are:

- the income statement which reports on income from and expenditure on the organization's regular operating activities during the accounting period;
- the balance sheet, which reveals the net assets of the organization at the end of the accounting period and the sources of funding of those assets;
- the cash flow statement, designed to reconcile the movement in cash balances to the performance as shown in the income statement.

Accountants use a number of concepts in preparing accounts. These include the accruals concept, the entity concept, the going concern concept, money measurement, consistency, materiality, conservatism and several others.

References

Buckley, M., Brindley, B. and Greenwood, M. (1997) *Business Studies*. London: Longman.

IASC (International Accounting Standards Committee) (2004) *Summary of individual International Accounting Standards 1 to 19 in force as of 1 January 2004*, http://www.iasb.org/standards/summary_ias01to19.asp, accessed 15 June 2004.

10 | The income statement

Overview

The next three chapters introduce the financial statements. In this chapter you will be concentrating on income and costs which are summarized in the income statement. As explained in Chapter 9, both the income and expenditure account and the profit and loss account refer to the same thing as the income statement, which is the term used in the IAS. However, income and expenditure is most often used in relation to not-for-profit organizations, the basis of most health care organizations. This chapter will give you the skills to read an income statement and identify the major sources of income and the major cost items as well as the ability to identify any significant changes in performance between the accounting period in question and the previous accounting period.

Learning objectives

By the end of this chapter you should be able to:

- **describe the purpose of an income statement**
- **identify the components of an income statement**
- **highlight issues for further exploration in an income statement**
- **consider the impact of alternative depreciation policies on reported financial performance**
- **identify the links between the income statement and the balance sheet**

Key terms

Accruals Expenses that the organization has incurred during the accounting period but for which invoices have not yet been received.

Depreciation The process of accounting for the reduction in value of an asset over the period of its useful life.

Net book value The historic or original cost of an asset minus accumulated depreciation to date.

Operating expenses The costs incurred by an organization in the course of its ordinary activities.

Operating income The income earned by an organization in the course of its ordinary activities.

Operating surplus (deficit) The difference between the operating income and operating expenses; a deficit will be incurred when expenses exceed the income.

Prepayments Payments made during the accounting period in respect of benefits which will be enjoyed in a future accounting period.

Reducing balance method A method of depreciation which assumes the greatest reduction in the value of an asset will be in the earliest years of its useful economic life; each accounting period depreciation is calculated as a percentage of the asset's net book value at the beginning of the accounting period.

Residual value The value at which an asset is considered likely to be sold at the end of its useful economic life.

Retained surplus (deficit) The surplus or deficit that remains after all expenses have been paid, interest payments on loans have been made and taxes and dividends, where applicable, have been paid.

Straight-line method A method of depreciation in which the estimated residual value is subtracted from the original cost of an asset and the depreciation is spread evenly over the useful economic life of that asset.

Useful economic life The period over which the owner of an asset will derive some economic benefit from its use.

The income statement

The income statement shows the organization's income and expenditure or costs relating to its activities for the accounting period. Its presentation is usually vertical and the layout generally follows the same standard pattern. The principal elements are shown in Table 10.1.

Table 10.1 Principal elements of an income statement

Income statement for the year ending [date]	
Operating income	A
less: operating expenses	B
Operating surplus (deficit)	A − B
less: overheads	C
less: interest, tax, dividends	D
Retained surplus (deficit)	A − B − (C + D)

Interest on loans, tax payable and dividends payable to stakeholders or funding agencies are optional items depending on the arrangements under which the organization operates. Some of these items are important for the distinction between private and public sector organizations. For example, dividends payable to shareholders and tax liability are characteristics of private sector organizations which are usually not relevant to the public sector. You should also note that the equivalent to surplus (deficit) in private organizations is profit (loss).

For any organization to survive in the long term, its income from operating activities should at least match and preferably exceed its expenditure. Table 10.2 shows a simple example of an income statement.

Table 10.2 Simple example of an income statement

	Note	This year ($000)	Last year ($000)
Gross income	1	100	80
Operating expenses	2, 3, 4	(65)	(82)
Operating surplus		35	(2)
Extraordinary items	5	(10)	2
Operating surplus/(deficit) before interest		25	nil
Interest	6	(3)	(3)
Surplus/(deficit) on ordinary activities		22	(3)

Note that in financial statements parentheses or brackets are used to indicate a negative. So in the account above $65,000 is to be subtracted from the $100,000 gross income and any total or subtotal which appears in parenthesis indicates a deficit, that is, that expenses exceeded income.

The numbers in the 'notes' column refer the reader of the accounts to further details on these headings that can be found in the notes that are attached to the accounting statements. By looking up Note 1 to the example accounts in Table 10.2 you would be able to discover the sources of the organization's income. Similarly, Notes 2 and 3 would provide a breakdown of the operating expenses. The operating expenses total will be adjusted in line with the accruals concept by deducting from them any *prepayments* in respect of subsequent accounting periods and adding to them any *accruals* for expenses that the organization has incurred but for which it has not yet been billed. So, these first two lines summarize the financial results of carrying out the activity for which the organization is established (its ordinary operating activities). The extraordinary items heading refers to income generated or costs incurred in carrying out exceptional transactions and would, for example, include the costs of restructuring the organization and closing down one area of activity, or selling off unwanted premises at a profit to the organization. The interest heading refers to interest paid to the organization on deposits held at the bank and on other investments as well as to interest paid on loans including bank overdrafts.

Activity 10.1

Turn to the latest accounts for the organization for which you work and locate the income statement. Read this carefully, referring to the notes to the accounts if necessary, in order to answer the following questions.

Note that the terminology and format of presentation may be slightly different from that used here but you should nevertheless be able to identify the required information. If you are unable to obtain a set of accounts for your own organization you may instead refer to the Someplace Hospital Annual Accounts for the year ended 31 March 2004, which you will find in Appendix 1 to this book. You should note that the Someplace

Accounts have been drawn up for a fictitious private hospital, so the layout and terminology probably won't match those of your organization's accounts. However, using these accounts will help you understand the generic format of an income statement and provide an insight into the differences between private and public sector organizations. If you are working in the public sector, you will find that some of the features of the accounts such as tax and dividend payments will probably not appear in your organization's income statement. Of course it is not possible to provide customized feedback to the activities, so feedback is instead given on the Someplace Hospital accounts.

1   What was the operating surplus (or deficit)/profit (or loss) for the year? What was the operating surplus (or deficit)/profit (or loss) for the previous year?
2   Find out the sources of income from the various activities.
3   What was the most significant operating expense item? Was this higher or lower than for the previous year?

Feedback

Your answers will be unique to the organization whose accounts you examined. The answers for Someplace Hospital are as follows:

1   The operating profit for the year ended 31 March 2004 was $1,011,000. The operating profit for the previous year was $1,229,000. (Someplace is a private hospital running on a for-profit basis.)

2   This information was included in Note 3 to the accounts of Someplace Hospital: the main sources of income were the government and insurance schemes, other sources were private patients and an unspecified 'other' category.

3   Staff costs of $38,431,000 were the most significant expense item. In the previous year staff costs amounted to $34,222,000 (Note 4).

Operating expenses

As you would expect, the most significant expense item for most health services is staff costs. The operating expenses total will also include clinical and general supplies and services, costs of maintaining premises and equipment, and transport costs, all of which have been incurred in the daily operations of the service.

In addition, there may be an amount included in respect of 'bad debts'. If it becomes clear that there is no chance of recovering a particular debt owed to the organization, the debt is 'written off' and recognized as an expense in the annual accounts. Depending on the degree of risk that the organization will have to write off bad debts in the future, it may make a 'provision for bad debts'. Each year it will review its debtors and decide whether it should increase or decrease the level of provision for bad debts. An increase in the provision for bad debts will be included as an expense item in the income statement, while a reduction in the provision for bad debts will be included as a negative expense item, in effect reducing the organization's total expenses for the year.

You may also find that operating expenses includes costs in respect of clinical negligence claims or insurance premiums for clinical negligence. In some accounts you will find a provision for clinical negligence.

Depreciation

The concept of depreciation was briefly mentioned in Chapter 9. A fixed asset is one that has a long life and is acquired with a view to retaining it within the organization (it is not bought for resale). Fixed assets provide the infrastructure of an organization and the vast majority of them, such as equipment, motor vehicles, beds and office fittings may need to be replaced at some future date. The matching and accruals concept requires that the cost of using resources be accounted for, not when they are initially acquired but over the period of their useful lives. The process of accounting for the diminution in the value of fixed assets is known as *depreciation* and the process of accounting for the use of intangible assets, such as software licences, is known as *amortization*.

Terms that you will come across in relation to depreciation include:

- *the useful economic life of assets:* the period over which the present owner will derive some economic benefit from their use;
- *residual value:* the value at which the asset is considered likely to be sold at the end of its useful economic life;
- *net book value:* the historic or original cost of the asset minus accumulated depreciation to date. This is the value of assets that will appear in the balance sheet.

The organization must decide on an appropriate basis for depreciating its fixed assets. The most common methods of depreciation in use are:

1 The *straight-line method*, in which the estimated residual value is subtracted from the original cost of the asset and the depreciation is spread evenly over the useful economic life of that asset. Catering equipment costing $10,000 is expected to have a useful economic life of five years and will have an estimated residual value of $1000 after five years. Using the straight-line method, depreciation is calculated as follows:

$$\text{Depreciation per year} = \frac{\$10,000 - \$1000}{5} = \$1800 \text{ per year.}$$

2 The *reducing balance method* assumes that the greatest reduction in the value of the asset will occur in the earliest years of its useful economic life. Thus depreciation is calculated by applying a percentage rate to the asset's net book value at the beginning of the year:

Depreciation for the year = net book value at the start of the period × depreciation rate.

Activity 10.2

A community outreach project has bought a fleet of new vehicles at a cost of $100,000. It is estimated that the vehicles will have a useful life of three years and a residual value of $10,000.

1 Using:

a) the straight-line method of depreciation
b) the reducing balance method (depreciation rate = 54 per cent per annum),

calculate the annual depreciation charge for each year and complete Tables 10.3 and 10.4.

Table 10.3 Depreciation using the straight-line method

	Year 1 ($)	Year 2 ($)	Year 3 ($)
Annual depreciation charge			
Original cost			
Accumulated depreciation			
Net book value			

Table 10.4 Depreciation using the reducing balance method

	Year 1 ($)	Year 2 ($)	Year 3 ($)
Annual depreciation charge			
Original cost			
Accumulated depreciation			
Net book value			

2 Consider and write brief notes on the different impacts these methods will have on the income statement.

 Feedback

1 Your completed tables should be as in Tables 10.5 and 10.6.

2 The straight-line depreciation method will reflect a constant depreciation charge over the useful life of the asset, whereas under the reducing balance method the depreciation charge will be much higher and therefore be a greater drain on surplus in the early years of the asset's useful life. Depreciation is a significant expense item in the

Table 10.5 Depreciation using the straight-line method

	Year 1 ($)	Year 2 ($)	Year 3 ($)
Annual depreciation charge	30 000	30 000	30 000
Original cost	100 000	100 000	100 000
Accumulated depreciation	30 000	60 000	90 000
Net book value	70 000	40 000	10 000

accounts of most health services and the method used to calculate depreciation has an impact on the surplus or deficit in the income statement.

Table 10.6 Depreciation using the reducing balance method

	Year 1 ($)	Year 2 ($)	Year 3 ($)
Annual depreciation charge	54 000	24 840	11 426
Original cost	100 000	100 000	100 000
Accumulated depreciation	54 000	78 840	90 266
Net book value	46 000	21 160	9 734

Note that the consistency concept applies equally to depreciation policies so that organizations cannot suddenly decide to change the method of depreciation that they use. The going concern concept allows the accountant to use depreciation to spread the cost of tangible assets over their useful economic lives.

In most published accounts you will find a statement of accounting policies. This statement is likely to make some reference to the depreciation methods used and to the agreed useful life of fixed assets. Office computers, because they are likely to become outdated very quickly, are, for example, likely to have a far shorter useful economic life than say, X-ray equipment, which may be in use for ten years or more.

It is one of the duties of the auditors to satisfy themselves that the methods of depreciation used are appropriate and that the net book value of assets, as shown in the balance sheet, is a true and fair reflection of their value as at the balance sheet date.

Activity 10.3

1 Turn to the accounts for the organization where you work or to the Someplace Hospital accounts and find:

    a) the depreciation for the year on the various categories of fixed assets
    b) an explanation of the organization's depreciation and amortization policies.

2 Spend a few minutes comparing the income statement of your organization with those of Someplace Hospital. Note the main differences in the headings and terminology.

Feedback

1 The depreciation detail for the year will be found in the notes to the accounts, although it may be included in a note relating to the tangible assets as listed in the balance sheet rather than as a note to the income statement. In the Someplace Hospital accounts, the depreciation is included in Note 11, the schedule of tangible fixed assets. If you were unable to find a statement regarding depreciation and amortization policies

you may wish to speak to one of the financial accountants in the organization and ask them what depreciation methods they use. You should, in any case, refer to Note 1.2, Statement of Accounting Policies, to the accounts of Someplace Hospital, which explains the basis of depreciation for various categories of assets and details the standard asset lives used in depreciating equipment, and Note 1.3, which describes the accounting treatment of intangible fixed assets.

2 If you work in a public sector organization you are likely to have found several differences in terminology on the income statement. These will arise from the fact that Someplace is a private hospital operating for profit. You may find references to surplus or deficit in place of references to profit or loss. You may also find no reference to tax or to dividends on the income statement of your organization. Depending on their residual claimant status, public sector organizations may not be liable for tax. Similarly, all surplus earnings may be retained or accumulated as part of the organization's accumulated fund, whereas private organizations may distribute a share of the profits to the owners in the form of dividends.

Profit or loss on disposal of fixed assets

The income statement includes a separate entry showing the profit or loss on the disposal of fixed assets. When fixed assets are sold off they are written out of the accounts at their net book value – cost less depreciation. However, the price obtained is very rarely the same as the net book value. The difference between the net book value and the proceeds of the sale of the asset is treated as a profit (or loss) on the disposal of fixed assets.

Tax

Someplace Hospital is a private hospital and pays tax on the profits it earns. The residual claimant status of health care organizations determines their tax liability. You will remember investigating the residual claimant status of your organization in Chapter 1.

Dividends

As discussed in Chapter 1, many organizations in the health sector operate as not-for-profit organizations and reinvest any surplus income. However, at the discretion of the directors, organizations that operate for profit will distribute a share of their profit to shareholders in the form of dividends. Dividend payments are rarely used in public sector organizations. An exception is the British NHS where hospital trusts are expected to return a 3.5 per cent dividend on capital to government (the owner).

Retained earnings

Retained earnings is the surplus or profit that remains after all expenses have been paid, interest payments on loans have been made and taxes and dividends where applicable have been paid. If an organization does not distribute its profit it can retain it to finance further expansion. Retained profit is one of the most significant sources of funding in the private sector but may be less so for organizations that do not set out to make a profit or surplus.

Recognized gains and losses

Before moving on to study the balance sheet in the next chapter, it is important to recognize the distinction between the increase in capital and reserves and the surplus as stated in the income statement. During the year, fixed assets such as land and buildings may be revalued. However, the potential gain cannot be included in the profit unless the property has been sold and the gain has been realized. The increase in value may, however, be included in the value of fixed assets on the balance sheet and credited to a revaluation reserve, in effect treating the increase in value as an increase in the organization's capital. In addition to donations and grants received on a regular basis for operating purposes, health care organizations may also receive substantial assets that have either been donated or financed by government grants. These, too, should be credited to a reserve account.

A statement of total recognized gains and losses takes account of the increases and any decreases in reserves, adding them to the surplus or deficit for the year to obtain the total recognized gains in the financial year. However, a 'statement of changes in equity' as recommended by the International Accounting Standards Board (IASB) may be included in the financial statements in place of the statement of total recognized gains and losses.

Summary

The income statement summarizes the organization's financial performance over the accounting period. With some differences in terminology, the format of the income statement is as follows: first, operating surplus (or deficit) is calculated by deducting operating expenses from all operating income. Then any one-off or unusual income or expenditure is included, to arrive at a surplus (or deficit) before interest. Next, interest receivable is added and interest payable is deducted leaving the surplus (or deficit) for the financial year. Finally any tax payable and dividends paid will be deducted, leaving the retained surplus (or deficit) for the year.

Depreciation is the mechanism used to account for the use of resources, not when they are initially acquired but over the period of their useful lives. The choice of method of depreciation can have a significant impact on the level of reported profits.

Any surplus income after the payment of tax (if applicable) and the distribution of dividends is retained and is reflected on the balance sheet along with accumulated surpluses from previous years. Retained earnings is often the most significant source of capital.

The balance sheet

Overview

In this chapter you will be concentrating on the balance sheet. The balance sheet shows what assets the organization owns and how these are funded. This chapter will give you the skills to read and analyse a balance sheet and to identify the links between the income statement and the balance sheet.

Learning objectives

By the end of this chapter you should be able to:

- **state the purpose of a balance sheet**
- **identify the components of the balance sheet**
- **read a balance sheet so as to determine the net worth of an organization and how it has been funded**
- **identify and explain the links between the income statement and the balance sheet**

Key terms

Current assets Short-term resources either held in the form of cash or expected to become cash within the next 12 months.

Current liabilities Amounts due for payment within 12 months from the balance sheet date.

Fixed assets Assets acquired for continuing use within the organization with a view to enabling it to carry out its normal operations.

Long-term liabilities Amounts due for payment more than 12 months after the balance sheet date.

Reserves Funds theoretically due to the owners but which have been retained within the organization for some reason; the most common reserves are retained surplus or profit.

Share capital Funds that have been invested in an organization by its shareholders.

Shareholders' funds The share capital and reserves of an organization.

Working capital (net current assets) Current assets minus current liabilities; this is the capital that is used in day-to-day operations.

What is a balance sheet?

The balance sheet and the income statement are the summary financial statements showing the state of affairs of the organization at a particular date and how the organization has performed over a period of time.

- The balance sheet shows what financial resources are available and where the money comes from. It is often referred to as a snapshot of a business since it reflects its financial standing at a particular moment. In theory the moment is midnight on the last day of the accounting period.
- The income statement, or profit and loss account, shows what return is being generated from these assets.

This information can be used to look at past performance or to look ahead and set performance targets for the future by adjusting the accounts to reflect future plans.

As you have seen in Chapter 9, a simple balance sheet (as in the statements of affairs, Tables 9.1 to 9.3) lists capital, liabilities and assets. However, such a basic version would not take account of the time frame during which assets are employed or when liabilities become due. So on a balance sheet the distinction is made between current and long-term (or fixed) assets and between current and long-term liabilities. These categories will be discussed later in this chapter.

In Chapter 9 the accounting equation, assets = capital + liabilities was introduced. Table 11.1 shows the elements contained in a balance sheet and the way in which they are usually presented. In this format the assets employed (A + D) will always equal the capital employed (E + F + G).

Table 11.1 Balance sheet outline

Fixed assets		A
Current assets	B	
Current liabilities	C	
Working capital (Current assets – current liabilities)	(B – C)	D
Assets employed		**A + D**
Financed by		
Long-term liabilities		E
Capital		F
Reserves		G
Capital employed		**E + F + G**

Note that here 'Capital employed' is the sum of:

long-term liabilities + capital + any reserves or retained profits

The accounting equation remains the same; it has been rearranged so that current liabilities – money that falls due for repayment within the next 12 months – is deducted from current assets and is not included in long-term liabilities. The reason for presenting current assets and liabilities in this way is that it makes it easy to calculate the value of the working capital, a concept that you will consider in Chapter 13.

Overall, the net assets employed are financed by the capital plus the long-term liabilities plus the reserves (funds due to owners) that have been retained within the organization for any of a number of reasons – see the section on balance sheet terms below.

Table 11.2 shows a simplified example of a balance sheet. If you look at the figures you can see the principles on which a balance sheet works. You may have noticed that in Table 11.2 long-term liabilities have been treated slightly differently from the way they were treated in Table 11.1. The long-term liabilities total has been subtracted from assets employed to give a 'total net assets' figure. This is, however, only a variation in presentation; the accounting equation remains unchanged. (In terms of Table 11.1, the equation becomes $A + D - E = F + G$.) You may come across either presentation in financial statements.

Table 11.2 Simplified balance sheet

Balance Sheet as at 30 September 2003

	Note	30 September 2003 $000	30 September 2003 $000	30 September 2002 $000	30 September 2002 $000
Fixed Assets					
Intangible assets	5	10		10	
Tangible assets	6	65		62	
			75		72
Current assets					
Stock	7	40		35	
Debtors:					
Trade	8	13		15	
Prepayments	9	2		3	
Cash at bank and in hand	10	5		4	
			60		57
Current liabilities					
Creditors amounts falling due within one year:					
Suppliers	11	(35)		(33)	
Accruals	12	(2)		(2)	
Bank overdraft		(10)		(11)	
			(47)		(46)
Net current assets (working capital)			13		11
Assets employed			88		83
Long-term liabilities			(15)		(15)
Total net assets			**73**		**68**
Financed by:					
Capital employed					
Capital	13		53		53
Reserves	14		20		15
Total capital employed			**73**		**68**

You will have seen that, as in the income statement, the balance sheet includes comparative figures for the previous year. It also includes references to supporting notes that provide further detail on various items within it.

The important thing to observe is that the balance sheet summarizes the assets owned and how they were financed. You can check this for yourself, by looking at the figures for 2003:

- total net assets $73,000 = capital employed $73,000

This equation can be expanded further:

- fixed assets $75,000 + current assets $60,000 – current liabilities $47,000 = capital $53,000 + reserves $20,000 + long-term liabilities $15,000

So you can see from this that whatever resources an organization has, these come from either outside the organization (current and long-term liabilities) or from the owners (the amounts included under capital and reserves). (The balance sheet of public sector organizations may not refer to 'capital' but instead to an accumulated fund.)

The other key thing to note is that the owners and the organization are treated as *separate and independent from each other*, so that, just as the organization recognizes what it owes for any loans or long-term liabilities, the organization is regarded as owing its owners whatever is due to them, either capital originally invested in the organization or reserves created from profit/surplus.

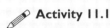 **Activity 11.1**

The following questions will help you to check your understanding of the purpose of a balance sheet.

1 Describe a balance sheet in one sentence.
2 What is the main difference between an income statement and a balance sheet?

 Feedback

Compare your answers with the following:

1 A balance sheet is a statement showing the assets, liabilities and capital of an organization at a particular moment.

2 An income statement summarizes income and expenditure over a period of time while a balance sheet reflects the state of affairs at a given moment.

Balance sheet terms

Some of the terms in the simplified balance sheet in Table 11.2 may have been unfamiliar to you. The following brief explanation may help, though the notes to the accounts are usually fairly easy to understand.

Assets

Assets are valuable resources that are owned by the organization. For financial accounting purposes, assets are regarded as either fixed or current.

Fixed assets

Fixed assets are assets acquired for continuing use within the organization with a view to enabling it to carry out its normal operations. Fixed assets are not normally bought with a view to resale. They include long-term investments, land, buildings, machinery, vehicles and equipment. Fixed assets are usually stated on the balance sheet at original cost less accumulated depreciation. However, where the value of land and buildings has significantly increased over a period of years, it may be decided to show their increased value on the balance sheet, with the balancing entry being an increase in the reserves under the capital employed heading.

Fixed assets are classified as either tangible or intangible.

- *Intangible assets* are not physical assets but nevertheless enable the organization to carry out its normal activities. Examples in the case of health services are software licences for computer systems and the results of research and development. These may be written off or amortized over the period of a licence or an agreed number of years in the case of research and development.
- *Tangible assets*, on the other hand, are assets having a physical identity, such as land, buildings, plant and machinery.

Note that staff, although regarded as the most valuable resource in many health care organizations, are not assets because they are not owned by the organization and because under the money measurement concept it is not possible to put a monetary value on their expertise.

Current assets

Current assets are short-term resources either held in the form of cash or expected to become cash within the next 12 months. On the balance sheet the three main current assets appear in reverse order of liquidity. They are:

- stocks, which in health care organizations may include supplies of drugs and dressings, X-ray film, office stationery and cleaning materials;
- debtors, people or organizations who owe money for goods or services provided and whose debts are payable within the next 12 months;
- cash in hand and cash at the bank in current and short-term savings accounts.

To the debtors total will be added any *prepayments* – expense items relating to the next accounting period that have been paid in advance. Typically these will include rental and insurance premiums. If part of the benefit has already been received, then only the portion relating to the next year will be regarded as a prepayment.

Liabilities

A liability is money which is owed to another. Liabilities are classified as either current or long term.

Current liabilities

Current liabilities are due for payment within 12 months from the balance sheet date and often much sooner. They include trade creditors who are owed payment for goods or services provided, taxation where applicable and bank overdrafts.

To current liabilities will be added *accruals* – any amounts due for which payment has not yet been requested. An example of an accrual is a telephone or electricity bill that is expected but has not yet been received.

The total of current liabilities is deducted from the total of current assets to obtain a total referred to as *working capital*, or net current assets. It is important that an organization is able to meet its short-term liabilities from its short-term assets, otherwise it would have to sell off valuable fixed assets to do so. Therefore, as you will see in Chapter 13, a great deal of importance is placed on the level of working capital as shown on the balance sheet.

Long-term liabilities

Amounts that a company has borrowed and which it must pay back more than 12 months after the balance sheet date are long-term liabilities. These would include long-term loans and mortgages.

The distinction between short-term and long-term liabilities in the balance sheet is important because, to maintain financial stability, organizations should ensure that they are in a position to meet their debt obligations when they arise. So, assets which will be held for a long period of time such as land and buildings should be financed by long-term sources of finance such as mortgages. Using short-term finance to fund the purchase of fixed assets may mean the organization will not be able to repay the debt when it becomes due and may be forced to sell assets in order to meet its obligations.

Capital

Capital is funds that have been invested in the organization by its owners. In the private sector, such investment is normally raised through shares sold to investors. In the public or not-for-profit sectors, investment may come from the state, charitable funds or other sources.

Reserves

Reserves are funds theoretically due to owners but which may be retained within the organization for a variety of reasons. They include:

• revaluation reserves where, as mentioned above, assets have been revalued to reflect their increased value;

- income and expenditure reserves, also referred to as retained surplus or retained profit;
- donation or endowment reserves, which include donations made for specific purposes.

The total of capital and reserves is referred to as total *equity*, where equity is defined as net assets of an entity after all creditors have been paid.

What can a balance sheet tell you?

Activities 11.2 and 11.3 will not only familiarize you with the terms discussed here but will also give you some insights into the financial standing of the organization as at the date of the balance sheet.

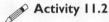 **Activity 11.2**

To check your understanding of these balance sheet terms, say which term describes each of the following:

- a mortgage negotiated to finance the building of a new clinic
- drugs
- an ultrasound scanner
- a pediatrician
- money on deposit at the bank
- an insurance premium that has been paid up for the next year
- an IT system
- power consumed but for which a bill has not yet been received
- money due within the next six months in respect of health care contracts for services delivered up to and including the balance sheet date

 Feedback

You should have classified the items as follows:

- a mortgage negotiated to finance the building of a new clinic – long-term liabilities
- drugs – current assets, stock
- an ultrasound scanner – tangible fixed assets
- a pediatrician – staff members do not appear in the balance sheet
- money on deposit at the bank – current assets, cash
- an insurance premium that has been paid up for the next year – current assets, prepayments
- an IT system – the hardware is a tangible fixed asset, software licences are intangible fixed assets
- power consumed but for which a bill has not yet been received – short-term liabilities, accruals
- money due within the next six months in respect of health care contracts – current assets, debtors

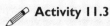

Activity 11.3

Refer to the balance sheet for your organization and answer the following questions. You will probably also need to refer to the notes to the accounts to find the answers to some of the questions. If you are unable to obtain a balance sheet for your organization, refer to the Someplace Hospital accounts in Appendix 1.

1   Was there any significant difference in fixed assets between the current year's and the previous year's balance sheet dates?
2   What was the working capital figure as at the balance sheet date?
3   What long-term liabilities does the organization have?
4   How are the net assets of the organization financed?
5   What was the organization's surplus (or deficit) for the year?

Feedback

Your answers will be unique to your organization. If you look at the Someplace Hospital accounts you may note the following.

1 Over the year the value of fixed assets fell from $14,110,000 to $10,721,000. If you look at Note 11 to the accounts you will see that this is referred to as 'net book value'. Net book value in this case is equal to the original cost of the asset less accumulated provisions for depreciation over the life of the asset to date. You will see from Note 11 to the accounts that any change in tangible fixed assets will also reflect disposals and acquisitions, that is, fixed assets sold and bought, during the year.

2 The working capital figure on 31 March 2004, the end of the Someplace Hospital accounting period, was $17,064,000.

3 The balance sheet shows that Someplace Hospital has long-term liabilities (shown as creditors – amounts falling due after more than one year) of $7,798,000. Note 15 to the accounts explains that the hospital has taken out a loan to finance the building of a new hospital wing.

4 The net assets of Someplace Hospital are financed by share capital, with revaluation and income and expenditure reserves.

5 The surplus (deficit)/profit (loss) for the year is not stated on the balance sheet but is included in the income and expenditure reserve total of $5,213,000. Note 17 details the movements on reserves and shows that a profit of $177,000 was transferred from the income statement. You should have recognized this as the retained profit for the year shown in the income statement.

If you found a significant increase in fixed assets were you able to identify how they were financed? Was there a corresponding increase in long-term liabilities or in capital and reserves? It is unwise for organizations to use short-term debt to fund fixed assets because the repayment period will be far shorter than the useful life of the asset.

You will be returning to the question of the acceptable level of working capital in Chapter 13.

Links between income statement and balance sheet

Question 5 of Activity 11.3 should have helped you to view retained surplus (or deficit) as a link between the income statement and the balance sheet. The other link that you may have noted is depreciation, which is shown both as an expense on the income statement (to be found in the note detailing operating expenses) and as a reduction in the net book value of fixed assets (to be found in the schedule of tangible fixed assets note to the balance sheet). Amortization of intangible assets such as software licences and increases or reductions in provisions such as the provision for doubtful debts will also be included both under operating expenses in the income statement and in the notes explaining the summary figures shown on the balance sheet.

Now that you have some practical experience of reading a balance sheet, in the next chapter you will move on to the third financial statement, the cash flow statement.

Summary

The balance sheet summarizes the values of the assets and liabilities of an entity at a point in time, usually the last day of the accounting period. From a balance sheet it can be seen that assets – liabilities = capital.

The items included on the balance sheet include fixed assets that will be used by the organization over the long term. Current assets include stocks, debtors and cash. The sum of current assets less current liabilities (mainly trade creditors and bank overdraft) is referred to as working capital. Long-term liabilities are loans and other liabilities payable in more than one year's time. The total assets employed figure on the balance sheet will be equal to the owners' capital and any reserves.

Retained surpluses and provisions for depreciation, amortization and various contingencies are all to be found in both the income statement and the balance sheet.

12 The cash flow statement

Overview

In this chapter the focus is on the cash flow statement – the statement that explains the change in cash balances from one balance sheet date to the next, in terms of the cash flows into and out of the organization. In Chapter 9 you learned of the need for a cash flow statement and the general format it follows. This chapter will give you the skills to understand and analyse a cash flow statement. The chapter draws on the key terms introduced in Chapters 9 to 11.

Learning objectives

By the end of this chapter you should be able to:

- **state the purpose of a cash flow statement**
- **identify, in general terms, the components of a cash flow statement**
- **read a cash flow statement so as to determine the reasons for any significant change in the organization's liquidity position**

Cash flows

Over the lifetime of most business organizations, cash flows occur as a result of:

- initial capitalization, when either public or private sector funds are raised to finance the organization;
- capital programmes, when further capital is introduced or long-term loans raised to finance the acquisition of additional capital assets in the form of land, buildings, machinery, equipment and so on, and cash is used to pay for such acquisitions;
- the purchase of stocks and supplies for resale or use in providing services;
- the sale of goods and the provision of services, which generate cash but also use cash, for example, staff costs.

These cash flows are illustrated in Figure 12.1. You will notice two distinct areas in the figure:

- the lower part of the figure shows the flows of share capital and long-term loans, which fund the initial establishment of the organization and may finance its further expansion; related to these flows are cash flows arising from the purchase and sale of fixed assets;
- the upper part of the figure shows the working capital cycle in which cash is used to pay suppliers of goods and services and to purchase stock; services

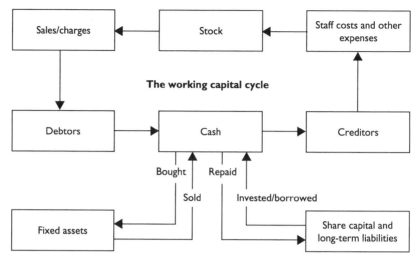

Figure 12.1 Organizational cash flows

and stocks are translated into sales which result in debtors from whom cash is duly received.

An organization's survival depends not so much on its ability to generate a surplus of income over expenditure, as on its ability to pay its debts when they are due. Cash is often referred to as the lifeblood of an organization, for without cash an organization would be unable to meet its commitments and in the longer term would be forced to cease operating. It is not surprising, therefore, that stakeholders of an organization will want to reassure themselves that the cash position is sound. For this reason it is usually required that a funds flow or cash flow statement should form part of the financial statements.

What is a cash flow statement?

Activity 12.1 will help you to recall the essence of the cash flow statement.

 Activity 12.1

Use what you have learnt in Chapters 9 to 11 to explain why an organization that has a substantial surplus of income over expenditure may end the year with less cash in hand and at the bank than at the beginning of the year.

 Feedback

Two possible explanations might be:

1 Accruals accounting requires income to be entered into the accounts for the period when it was earned even though the cash may not yet have been received, thus a surplus

or profit may be shown even though the cash at hand is lower than the previous year. (The debtors balance would include such amounts owing to the organization.)

2 The income statement shows only income and expenditure arising from ordinary operational activities. Therefore the purchase of an expensive capital item would not be reflected in the income statement although it would cause a reduction in the level of cash and bank balances.

The cash flow statement shows all of the cash payments and cash receipts in the accounting period. Its layout is prescribed within the accounting standards framework. Table 12.1 shows the usual headings in a cash flow statement, and indicates the activities where inflow and outflow of cash may arise.

Table 12.1 Elements of cash flow statements

Activity/heading	Inflow	Outflow
1 Net cash inflow (outflow) from operating activities	From customers	To staff and suppliers
2 Returns on investment and servicing of finance	Interest received	Interest and dividends paid
3 Taxation		Tax paid
4 Capital expenditure/ investing activities	Sale of fixed assets	Purchase of fixed assets
5 Dividends paid		To owners
6 Financing	New capital received New loans raised	Repayment of loans

Net cash inflow from operating activities

The first heading in a typical cash flow statement is the net cash inflow (outflow) from operating activities. This is a net figure and to find out how it was calculated, you will probably need to refer to a note to the accounts.

There are a number of items that appear in the income statement as income or expenditure but that do not actually give rise to cash flows. These include:

- income earned but not yet received (as described in Activity 12.1);
- transfers from reserves;
- depreciation and amortization charges (you saw in Chapter 10 that these are accounting entries only and do not involve the movement of cash);
- purchases on credit (the purchases are included in operating expenses), but until the creditors are paid the amount is reflected as an increase in the creditors shown on the balance sheet and no cash is paid.

Net cash inflow from operating activities is calculated by adjusting the operating surplus (or deficit) for such non-cash transactions. Tables 12.2 and 12.3 display two different scenarios with different directions and sizes of cash flows. They both show how the operating surplus figure is adjusted to calculate the net cash inflow (or outflow) from operating activities.

Table 12.2 Reconciliation of operating surplus to net cash inflow from operating activities

	Note	1 September 2003–31 August 2004 ($)	Information source
Operating surplus for the year		12 400	Income statement
Depreciation charges	1	23 482	Notes to the income statement
Amortization of software licences	1	2 500	Notes to the income statement
Decrease in stocks	2	5 000	Balance sheet
Decrease in debtors	3	8 000	Balance sheet
Increase in creditors	4	6 718	Balance sheet
Increase in provision for doubtful debts	5	1 500	Notes to the income statement
Net cash inflow from operating activities	6	59 600	

Notes:
1 Although depreciation and amortization are treated as operating expenses, they are book entries only and so there is no cash outflow. They are therefore added back onto the operating surplus for the year.
2 A reduction in the level of stocks or supplies held means that there is less cash 'tied up' whereas an increase in the level of stocks held would mean that more cash was tied up in stocks. So a decrease is added back to the operating surplus.
3 A reduction in the debtors' balances means that there is less money owed to the organization than at the end of the previous year, so this decrease should be added to the operating surplus. An increase in debtors' balances would have the opposite effect, so any increase should be subtracted from the operating surplus.
4 If there is an increase in the creditors' balances this means that the organization has not yet paid the cash it owes and its cash balances will be higher than if it had paid those creditors. An increase in the level of creditors should be added to an operating surplus but a decrease in the level of creditors should be subtracted from the operating surplus.
5 An increase in provision for doubtful debts is classified as an expense in the income statement but it does not involve any cash flow, so the increase should be added to the operating surplus. A reduction in the provision for doubtful debts should be subtracted from the operating surplus.
6 The net cash inflow (or outflow) from operating activities is the sum of all of the preceding figures; it is the first line of the cash flow statement.

Table 12.3 Reconciliation of operating surplus to net cash outflow from operating activities

	Note	1 September 2003–31 August 2004 ($)	Information source
Operating surplus for the year		12 400	Income statement
Depreciation charges	1	23 482	Notes to the income statement
Amortization of software licences	1	2 500	Notes to the income statement
(Increase) in stocks	2	(10 000)	Balance sheet
(Increase) in debtors	3	(18 000)	Balance sheet
(Decrease) in creditors	4	(9 718)	Balance sheet
(Decrease) in provision for doubtful debts	5	(1 500)	Notes to the income statement
Net cash inflow (outflow) from operating activities	6	(836)	

Notes:
1–5 As for Table 12.2.
6 In this case the reconciliation reflects a net cash outflow from operating activities.

Activity 12.2

Write a brief explanation, in point form, as to why Table 12.2 reflects a net cash inflow from operating activities while Table 12.3 reflects a net cash outflow from operating activities even though the operating surplus for the year was the same in both cases.

 Feedback

Although depreciation and amortization were the same in both cases, Table 12.3 shows that:

- both stocks and debtors' balances increased
- there was a reduction in the level of creditors
- there was a decrease in provision for doubtful debts

All of these meant that there was less cash flowing into the organization over the period than in the scenario given in Table 12.2.

Returns on investment and servicing of finance

The entry for returns on investment and servicing of finance is brought into the cash flow statement from the income statement. It is the net total of interest received and interest paid by the organization over the period.

Taxation

If the health service organization whose accounts you are studying pays tax then there will be an entry under this heading, with net tax paid during the period being subtracted from a net cash inflow.

Dividends paid

Similarly, not all health care organizations pay dividends but those that do will subtract the cash paid out in dividends (as shown in the income statement) from a net cash inflow from operating activities.

Capital expenditure/investing activities

The income statement includes only revenue transactions; it excludes capital transactions such as the purchase or sale of fixed assets and the repayment or raising of loans. Such transactions, which are summarized in the balance sheet (with detail provided in the supporting notes), can give rise to substantial cash flows and they have a very significant impact on the financial health of an organization.

Capital expenditure includes payments to acquire fixed assets and proceeds from the sale of fixed assets. Purchases represent an outflow of cash while proceeds from the sale of fixed asset are an inflow.

Financing

This final heading refers to capital movements and changes in long-term liabilities between balance sheet dates. Additional capital raised in the form of shares or long-term loans are inflows, while the redemption of shares and the repayment of long-term loans are cash outflows.

Where does the information come from?

The cash flow statement is supplementary to the income statement and the balance sheet in the sense that it uses information from these two statements to explain cash movements.

Activity 12.3 gives you the opportunity to check your understanding of this chapter by identifying the sources of the information that is included in the cash flow statement and reflecting on the effect that each type of transaction will have on cash balances.

 Activity 12.3

Table 12.4 outlines the main headings of a cash flow statement. Alongside each, note:

1 Whether the information would be found in the income statement or the balance sheet.
2 Whether this type of transaction would have a positive or negative effect on cash balances.

The first row has been filled in for you.

Table 12.4 The cash flow statement

	Information source	Effect on cash balances
Operating surplus (deficit) for the year	I & E or BS notes, this information appears on both	Surplus = positive, deficit = negative
Increase (decrease) in stocks		
Increase (decrease) in debtors		
Increase (decrease) creditors		
Interest received, interest paid		
Taxation paid (if relevant)		
Capital expenditure (acquisition of fixed assets)		
Disposal of fixed assets		
Dividends paid		
Increases in long-term loans		
Loan repayments		
Capital funding raised		

Feedback

Compare your completed table with Table 12.5.

Table 12.5 Cash flow statement analysis

	Information source	Effect on cash balances
Operating surplus (deficit) for the year	I & E or BS notes, this information appears on both	Surplus = positive, deficit = negative
Increase (decrease) in stocks	BS	Increased stocks = negative decreased stocks = positive
Increase (decrease) in debtors	BS	Increased debtors = negative decreased debtors = positive
Increase (decrease) creditors	BS	Increased creditors = positive decreased creditors = negative
Interest received, interest paid	Income statement	Interest received = positive interest paid = negative
Taxation paid (if relevant)	Income statement	Negative
Capital expenditure (acquisition of fixed assets)	BS notes	Negative
Disposal of fixed assets	BS notes	Positive
Dividends paid	Income statement	Negative
Increases in long-term loans	BS notes	Positive
Loan repayments	BS notes	Negative
Capital funding raised	BS notes	Positive

Reading a cash flow statement

The final activity of this chapter will give you practice in reading the cash flow statement of an organization. The cash flow statement for the organization in which you work may use a different format from the one discussed here. However, you should still be able to identify the required information.

Activity 12.4

Now return to the annual accounts for your organization or for Someplace Hospital and find the cash flow statement for the financial year you have been studying, along with the income statement and the balance sheet.

As you read the cash flow statement, trace the figures back to their sources in the income statement and the balance sheet. You will need to refer to the notes to the accounts and particularly the notes to the cash flow statement, in order to carry out this exercise. When you have done this, answer the following questions.

1   Was the cash at bank and in hand greater on the current or the previous year's balance sheet date?

2   Was the change in cash balances in the same direction and of the same size (more or less) as the net cash inflow from operating activities, i.e. after adjusting the operating surplus (or deficit) for depreciation, transfers from reserves and increases or decreases in stocks, debtors and creditors?

3   Aside from operating activities, what were the main cash flows into and out of the organization over the accounting period?

↻ Feedback

You should have been able to trace the source of each entry on the cash flow statement. If you had difficulty, then looking at the sources you identified in Activity 12.3 may help. Your answers will be unique to the accounts you studied. An analysis of Someplace Hospital's accounts reveals the following:

1   The balance sheet shows cash balances of $7,203,000 at the end of the period and of $4,714,000 at the beginning of the period – an increase of $2,489,000. This is the increase shown on the bottom line of the cash flow statement.

2   The net cash inflow from operating activities (Note 18.1 to the cash flow statement) was $127,000 while net cash actually increased by $2,489,000. This indicates that there were substantial cash inflows that were not related to operating activity.

3   The main inflows were from the sale of tangible fixed assets. Outflows were smaller in scale; the main outflows were payments to acquire both tangible and intangible fixed assets and dividends and tax paid. If you were to find such a situation in your organization's accounts you might wish to find out why fixed assets of this value had been sold. Were they merely surplus to requirements and will their sale affect the operating capability of the organization?

Now that you have some practical experience of reading financial statements, in the next two chapters you will move on to learn about the management of working capital and see how financial statements can be used to control and interpret organizational performance.

Summary

The cash flow statement reconciles the movement in cash balances between one balance sheet date and the next. Taking, as its starting point, the operating surplus, it adjusts this to reveal the net cash inflow from operating activities by adding back depreciation, which is a non-cash expense, and adjusting the surplus or deficit to take account of movements in debtors' and creditors' balances and stocks. The next step is to include cash movements as a result of interest receipts and payments, capital expenditure, taxation and dividend payments, and financing items such as loan receipts or repayments and capital movements. When all of these adjustments are made the remaining balance should equal the increase or decrease in cash as reflected on the balance sheet.

13 Working capital management

Overview

In this and the next chapter the focus will shift from reading and understanding financial statements to analysing and interpreting the information they contain, and using this information for management purposes. This chapter concerns an aspect of financial management that is revealed in the balance sheet – the management of working capital. You will examine its vital importance in the organizational context. This chapter will give you an understanding of the importance of working capital management and help you to identify what needs to be done to ensure that the working capital cycle is not interrupted. You will focus on cash forecasting and management techniques and learn about treasury management.

Learning objectives

By the end of this chapter you should be able to:

- **explain the importance of working capital management**
- **review the ways in which control of working capital, and especially cash, is exercised across the organization**
- **distinguish between income and receipts and between expenditure and payments**
- **prepare a simple cash forecast**

Key terms

Cash flow forecast (cash budgets) Budgets which profile cash flows over the budget period, to ensure that there is enough cash to meet operational and other needs.

Working capital cycle The cycle in which cash is used to pay creditors and also to pay staff and to purchase supplies, so enabling the organization to generate income from its operations which results either in immediate cash payments or in debtors who will, in due course, pay cash to settle their debts.

The importance of working capital

It is vitally important that managers are able to effectively manage working capital on an ongoing basis. For this, managers need their financial accounting system to generate regular, reliable and accurate reports that will provide them with the necessary information to do so.

You will remember from earlier chapters that working capital = current assets – current liabilities. Current assets include stocks of goods for resale and consumables, such as dressings, food stocks and cleaning materials, debtors and prepayments, and cash in hand and at the bank. Current liabilities are trade creditors who must be paid within the next 12 months, and bank overdrafts.

Figure 13.1 focuses on the *working capital cycle*, which was briefly introduced in Chapter 12. Cash is used to pay creditors and also to pay staff and to purchase supplies. The organization generates income from its operations and this results either in immediate cash payments or in debtors who will, in due course, pay cash to settle their debts.

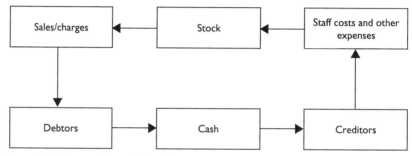

Figure 13.1 The working capital cycle

To ensure that operations run smoothly, every stage of the working capital cycle must be managed efficiently because:

- if there is insufficient cash to pay trade creditors they may withhold future supplies;
- cash must be available to pay salaries or staff will have to be released;
- an understaffed organization with inadequate supplies will be unable to meet demand for goods or services and sales/fee income will fall;
- this will lead to a further reduction in the level of cash balances and unless action is taken the downward spiral will continue.

Managing working capital

To ensure that there is enough cash to pay creditors when the amounts owing to them fall due, it is necessary to monitor and control every element of working capital on a regular and routine basis. The elements of working capital other than cash are now considered in turn. Managing cash is discussed later.

Stocks

Stocks are held in order to ensure that there are sufficient levels of physical resources available to meet operational needs. Depending on the nature of the service, health services may hold stocks of drugs, dressings, food, cleaning supplies, staff uniforms, linen etc. If stocks fall below a certain level the resulting shortages may cause delays in service delivery. On the other side of the coin, carrying too many stocks can have a number of adverse consequences: they can take up too much storage space; they may be held for so long that they become out of date and can no longer be used; and they tie up cash which might be used for other purposes. It is important for managers to strike a balance between holding stock 'just in case' it is needed in the future and buying in stock 'just in time' for it to be used (Mellett *et al.* 1993).

In recent years a rigorous approach to the management of supplies has been introduced as part of public sector reforms to many health care organizations. If you order drugs and medical supplies just when you need them ('just in time') you can make significant savings on space, energy and transportation. While this requires logistic skills and IT support, it saves costs by reducing the amount of resources tied up in the inventory and working capital. Even more important are quality improvements as contracts can be used to shift much of the responsibility for the quality of supplies from the provider to the supplier. Large health care organizations usually have the buying power to dominate the supplier network and impose common rules for quality assurance.

Reliable stock control procedures should be in place to ensure that:

• ordering systems are in place to ensure that stock is ordered at the right time;
• up-to-date stock records show both stocks received and stocks issued;
• there is a requisition procedure for the issuing of supplies from stock;
• stocks are kept appropriately – they are secure, there are no fire hazards, they are kept at the correct temperatures where necessary;
• regular stock counts confirm that stock records are correct.

Debtors

As you saw in Chapter 12, debtors represent cash that is owing to the business but has not yet been received. It makes sense, therefore, to keep the value of debtors as low as possible and to ensure that debtors settle promptly. While health services would probably find it difficult to operate on a purely cash basis, it is important that they carefully monitor the level of credit they are extending to debtors. In particular they should ensure that they are satisfied as to the prospective debtor's ability to pay the money they owe at an arranged future date. They should also ensure that the terms on which they are extending credit are made clear. All invoices and statements sent out to debtors should clearly state the number of days in which the debt must be settled.

As well as following the principles discussed above, the manager with responsibility for credit control should ensure that:

- invoices are issued promptly and that statements of account are sent out to debtors on a regular basis;
- a regular 'aged debtor analysis' is produced, showing the outstanding debts and the length of time for which they have been outstanding – this should be followed up with a determined effort to contact outstanding debtors;
- the amount tied up in debt is carefully monitored and any reasons for an increase in the debtors is understood (e.g. an increase may be because the level of operational activity and therefore of income has increased, or because debtors are being granted longer periods of credit);
- where, exceptionally, it is recognized that there is no chance of recovering a debt, the balance is removed from the debtor's ledger and written off to a bad debts account.

You should not, however, lose sight of the bigger picture: if it is possible to increase the level of activity in the short term then, by increasing income, you will increase the cash flows into the organization.

Prepayments

Prepayments include such items as annual insurance policies and rental payments made in advance. While in some cases these are standard practice, it should be recognized that, as with stock and debtors, they tie up funds that the organization might otherwise hold as cash, so they should be avoided where possible.

Creditors

Credit terms are often negotiated for the purchase of stocks and this is, in effect, a source of short-term finance to the organization. Two points are worth remembering:

- such credit may bear a cost in terms of discounts that may be offered by suppliers for cash settlement – in this case the discounts should be compared with the interest on cash balances that would be foregone if paying for goods at the time of purchase;
- managers must ensure that they have sufficient funds to meet these debts when they fall due – failure to settle outstanding debts may result in adverse credit terms in future and bad relations with suppliers.

Purchasing systems should be in place to ensure that only authorized purchases are made, that all goods and services for which the organization has been invoiced have in fact been received, and that accurate records are kept of payments made to creditors.

Accruals

You saw in Chapter 10 that accruals are costs which have been incurred even though the organization has not yet been invoiced for them. Utilities such as water and power are the most common examples. By monitoring usage, managers should be able to estimate accurately the amount of accruals.

Overdrafts

Bank overdrafts are a source of short-term finance. However, they are usually more expensive than other forms of finance so the level of bank overdraft should be carefully monitored.

Cash flow forecasts

Cash management is the most important aspect of working capital management. To be able to manage cash effectively, you need to be able to forecast cash flows. You saw in Chapter 8 that cash budgets, which profile cash flows over the budget period, ensure that there is enough cash to meet operational and other needs. Cash flow forecasts are an integral part of the budgeting process and they need to be monitored closely and kept up to date in the light of regular accounting reports of actual cash flows.

In drawing up a cash flow forecast, accountants will carefully consider the profile of the capital and revenue budgets for the organization to identify all of the associated cash receipts and payments and their timing. These will include:

- cash flows associated with the planned activities of the organization (such as fee and contract income, salaries and other staff costs, cash purchases, payments to creditors);
- payments for planned capital expenditure (staged payments for building projects, purchase of equipment, vehicles, computers etc.) and anticipated receipts from the disposal of fixed assets;
- cash flows associated with financing arrangements that are already in place (e.g. new loans that have been negotiated, loan repayments falling due, rental charges);
- all other cash flows such as tax and dividend payments and receipts from charitable sources.

Some of these flows, such as salaries, will be steady and regular, while others will be one-off. The most important point to note when preparing a cash forecast is that although income may be generated in one period, payment may not be received until much later.

The cash flow forecast prepared in association with the annual budget typically shows the level of cash at the beginning of a 12-month period and the forecast receipts and payments on a month-by-month basis, so that any shortfalls or surpluses can be predicted and plans put in place either to secure short-term finance or delay payments where possible or, in the case of surpluses, to ensure that surplus cash is invested at the best possible interest rate where it will be available when it is needed. Activity 13.1 will give you some understanding of how cash flow forecasts are drawn up.

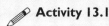

Activity 13.1

You are the financial manager of a rural health centre. The director of the health centre has asked you to prepare cash flow forecasts for the next four months. He is worried that the centre has insufficient funds in its bank account to cover the cost of building an extension. A loan has been arranged with the Ministry of Health but this will not meet the full cost of the building works.

The centre's only source of income is from providing health services to the local population on a fee-for-service basis. Patients do not always settle their bills at the time of treatment. Experience has shown that 60 per cent of payments are received in the same month as treatment and 30 per cent of payments are received in the month following treatment. The remaining 10 per cent are received in the second month after treatment.

Expenditure at the health centre consists of salaries and other costs (drugs, supplies and other running costs). Salaries are paid on the last Friday of the month and monthly expenditure on salaries is currently $22,000. All staff receive a 10 per cent pay rise on 1 May.

For other costs, experience shows that 70 per cent of bills are settled in the month of delivery and 30 per cent are settled during the following month.

Table 13.1 shows income and expenditure (other costs, not salaries) for March to June.

Table 13.1 Income and expenditure (other costs) March to June

Month	Income ($)	Expenditure (other costs) ($)
March	30 000	4 000
April	32 000	4 000
May	33 000	3 000
June	31 000	3 000

Income is estimated as $33,000 for January and $31,000 for February. Expenditure (other costs) is estimated as $4500 for February. The building works for the new extension will start on 12 March and are programmed to finish on 7 June. A contract price of $72,000 has been agreed for work and 10 per cent will be paid as a deposit on 5 March. Forty per cent is due by the end of April and 40 per cent by the end of May. The remaining 10 per cent is payable on completion of the contract.

The Ministry of Health's regional office is providing the health centre with a loan of $60,000 which will be deposited in the health centre's bank account on 1 April. The loan should be repaid in 24 equal instalments over the next four years – the first repayment being due on 31 May. In addition, the Ministry charges monthly interest of 1 per cent on the outstanding balance of the loan. Interest charges should be paid on the last day of each month and are payable from the month in which the loan is received.

Equipment costing $6000 will be purchased for the new extension in mid-April. The suppliers will allow 60 days' credit.

The cash balance at the beginning of March is $4250.

1 Prepare a cash flow forecast for the four months from March to June.
2 Estimate the debtors and creditors balances as at 30 June, making a note of how the loan for the extension would be treated on the balance sheet.

Remember that you need to think about the difference between income and cash flows. For example, for income relating to January, the actual cash receipts will not necessarily be received in January – some will be received in February and March.

Use Table 13.2 to help you in your calculations before entering your cash flow forecast in Table 13.3.

Table 13.2 Cash receipts and payments – workings

	Expected cash receipts ($)					
	March	*April*	*May*	*June*	*July*	*August*
Income relating to:						
January						
February						
March						
April						
May						
June						
July						
August						
Totals						

	Expected cash payments ($)					
	March	*April*	*May*	*June*	*July*	*August*
Expenditure (other costs) relating to:						
January						
February						
March						
April						
May						
June						
July						
August						
Totals						

Table 13.3 Cash flow forecast March to June

	March ($)	*April ($)*	*May ($)*	*June ($)*
Opening cash balance				
Add receipts:				
• Health care				
• Loan				
Less cash payments:				
• Salaries				
• Other costs				
• Building works				
• Equipment				
• Interest payment				
• Loan repayment				
Closing cash balance				

Feedback

1 Compare your completed cash flow forecast with the solution in Table 13.4.

Table 13.4 Cash flow forecast March to June (solution)

	March ($)	April ($)	May ($)	June ($)
Opening cash balance	4 250	1 500	37 400	10 400
Add receipts:				
• Health care	30 600	31 300	32 400	31 700
• Loan		60 000		
Less cash payments:				
• Salaries	22 000	22 000	24 200	24 200
• Other costs	4 150	4 000	3 300	3 000
• Building works	7 200	28 800	28 800	7 200
• Equipment				6 000
• Interest payment		600	600	575
• Loan repayment			2 500	
Closing cash balance	1 500	37 400	10 400	1 125

If you did not arrive at the same figures it may help to go carefully over the following workings.

Cash receipts (health care) for March are calculated as:

10 per cent of income for January (0.1 × $33,000 = $3300)
30 per cent of income for February (0.3 × $33,000 = $9300)
60 per cent of income for March (0.6 × $33,000 = $18,300)

Cash payments (other costs) for March are calculated as:

30 per cent of expenditure for February (0.3 × $4,500 = $1350)
70 per cent of expenditure for March (0.7 ×· $4000 = $2800)

2 Estimated debtors at 30 June are $15,700. This consists of:

$3300 of income relating to May for which payment will not have been received at 30 June
$12,400 of income relating to June for which payment will not have been received at 30 June

Estimated creditors at 30 June are $15,900. This consists of:

$900 (30 per cent of expenditure relating to June will not be paid until after June)
$15,000 in respect of loan repayments due within the next 12 months

The remaining balance of the loan ($42,500) would be regarded as a long-term liability and included as creditors (amounts falling due after more than one year).

Once the cash-flow forecast has been prepared it is possible to highlight potential times of cash shortage and to manage working capital in such a way as to minimize the requirement for short-term borrowing. Following up outstanding debtors, reviewing the level of stocks held so as to reduce purchases and negotiating longer credit terms from suppliers can all help to alleviate cash shortages.

Treasury management

It is usually the responsibility of the finance manager to ensure not only that there is enough cash to meet working capital requirements but also to ensure that:

- substantial sums of money are not left in accounts where they earn no interest – very large sums of money may even be invested overnight;
- short-term loan facilities such as overdrafts are in place and can be drawn on to meet short-term needs;
- appropriate long-term finance is negotiated to finance the acquisition of fixed assets.

To do this, finance managers will need a range of forecasts like the one you prepared in Activity 13.1, above, covering not only working capital but also the acquisition and disposal of fixed assets. Such forecasts will need to be broken down to provide weekly and in some cases even daily detail.

Summary

Working capital is equal to current assets less current liabilities. In the working capital cycle, cash is used to pay creditors and to meet staff costs and other expenses as well as to purchase stock. Staff use supplies in providing services for which charges are made. Debtors pay cash in respect of these charges. Each element must be carefully managed to ensure the organization is able to continue its operations.

Cash management involves carefully monitoring and controlling stock, debtors and creditors. To prepare a cash flow forecast you need to identify all income and expenditure for the period of the forecast, including income from and expenditure on capital assets. Then you must distinguish between income and receipts and between expenditure and payments, entering only the anticipated receipts and payments for each period.

Treasury management is concerned with ensuring that there are sufficient funds of the right kind to meet both working capital and long-term capital requirements and that those funds that will not be needed in the short term are invested to yield a return.

Reference

Mellett, H., Marriott, N. and Harries, S. (1993) *Financial Management in the NHS: A Manager's Handbook*. London: Chapman & Hall.

14 Interpreting financial statements

Overview

In Chapters 10 to 12 you learned how to read financial statements; in this chapter you will learn how to examine published accounts using the techniques of performance analysis to measure and quantify performance. The resulting ratios combine to present a powerful overview of financial performance. This overview can often be related to the business strategy and how successfully it is implemented. Because of the close links between strategy, operational performance and business planning, these ratios are used by chief executives, the board and senior executives to monitor and target organizational performance. Investigation of the ratios internally within the organization leads directly to the budgets and plans against which the actual divisional and departmental results are monitored. From this, corrective action is identified that will feed back into the results reported in the income and expenditure statements and balance sheets on which new updated performance ratios will be calculated.

Learning objectives

By the end of this chapter you should be able to:

- **explain the need for performance ratios**
- **identify performance ratios that provide information for different needs**
- **calculate performance ratios**
- **analyse and comment on performance using these performance ratios**

Key terms

Asset turnover The amount of income generated for each unit invested in fixed assets: income/average fixed assets.

Gearing (leverage) Indicator of whether an organization can meet its long-term liabilities; gearing is calculated as interest-bearing debt/non-interest bearing debt.

Liquidity (acid test) ratio A more critical test of an organization's ability to pay than the working capital ratio, the liquidity ratio excludes stock from the calculation, using cash + debtors/current liabilities.

Performance measures or ratios Techniques used to interpret financial statements.

Profit margin (operating margin) A measure of profitability: operating profit/surplus as a percentage of income.

Return on capital employed The return on capital invested in an organization calculated as profit before interest and tax/relevant net assets × 100.

Working capital ratio (current ratio) A measure that compares current assets with current liabilities to analyse the organization's ability to meet its short-term obligations; it is calculated as current assets/current liabilities.

Of what use to managers are financial statements?

As a management tool the financial statements introduced in Chapters 9 to 12 have a number of defects. Mellett *et al.* (1993) note the following limitations:

- they report activities which have already taken place and are therefore of little use for planning purposes;
- they contain only greatly summarized information;
- they show only absolute values that are not placed in any comparative context.

Financial statements, as you have already seen, are produced largely for an external audience. There may be times when you as a manager will want to refer to the financial reports of other organizations. You may, for example, wish to:

- compare your organization's performance with that of a close competitor;
- establish the financial standing of a prospective supplier to ensure that they will be able to continue to supply you;
- reassure yourself as to the liquidity position of a customer before agreeing credit terms;
- assess the viability of an organization with a view to an acquisition, merger or joint venture.

To overcome the problem of absolute values that are not placed in a comparative context, analysts have developed a series of financial ratios – measures based on figures in the financial statements that enable comparisons of performance and of liquidity.

Performance ratios

The question most people want answered when studying a set of accounts is: 'How well is the organization doing?' This is a very complicated question to answer and performance analysis will give you the skills to break down and analyse the financial components of performance.

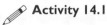 **Activity 14.1**

Before you go on to look at performance ratios there are several important things you need to understand. The way to understand these is to think of performance in terms of sporting activity. Imagine that you are a runner, perhaps even training competitively: how would you judge your performance? How would you know whether you were running well? Write down three or four of your ideas.

Feedback

> You should have plenty of ideas. An obvious one is to measure how many miles you can run in an hour or half an hour or whatever time interval you choose. This is a very sensible suggestion and it illustrates that performance measures compare one thing with another. Profit by itself or a net assets figure by itself does not tell you anything very helpful, but combine the two and you get a performance measure – return on capital employed, which compares profit with capital employed. It is the same for running: distance and time become more meaningful when combined.
>
> Then there are different ways of looking at performance measures. From an individual or internal perspective you would want to know how your running performance compared with previous occasions when you ran. For instance, have you beaten your personal record from last year? This internal perspective is the same for an organization. The trend in performance measures is important. So you can look at the performance measure this year and compare it with last year and note the trend in performance.
>
> But this is a highly individual or internal way of looking at performance. Despite an improving trend in your running you could enter the local marathon and come a disappointing last! It may be your own personal best but compared with other runners you are too slow and you know it. This is the other way of looking at performance externally, by comparing your running distance and times with other runners. It is the same for organizations, having compared performance measures or ratios internally to identify the trend, the same measures can be applied externally to compare performance with other organizations doing the same activities.

The techniques used to interpret financial statements can be divided into two broad categories:

- those dealing with the position as reflected in the balance sheet;
- those focusing on progress as reflected in the income statement and the cash flow statement.

Which performance ratios?

Using *performance ratios* is an art rather than a science. There are as many different ratios and approaches to calculating these as there are organizations that use ratios. So, if you read about ratios you will find many different explanations and options. By all means think about these and whether they can be of value to you in your organization. If you wish to introduce some of your own and the opportunity to do so is there, then that is to your advantage. But you can also do well by sticking to and using the ratios provided for you in this chapter. These are more than enough for a thorough and very sound analysis.

There are many different ways that performance can be analysed. Accounting ratios fall into three types:

- those that explore the financial position by analysing the structure and balance of assets and liabilities as shown on the balance sheet;

- those that analyse financial progress as shown in the income statement;
- combined ratios, which use data from both balance sheet and income statement.

A word about terminology

When you are learning to use accounting ratios one of the most confusing things can be differences in the terminology that is used in different sets of accounts. Throughout this chapter you will be using the accounts of both your own organization and of Someplace Hospital, included in Appendix 1. The next activity will help to familiarize you with the terminology used and to reconcile any apparent differences.

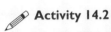 **Activity 14.2**

Using the Someplace Hospital accounts to guide you, see if you can find the direct counterpart, or equivalent term, in your own organization. For the items listed from the Someplace Hospital accounts in Table 14.1, write the equivalent item description for your own organization.

Table 14.1 Financial statement terminology

Someplace Hospital	Equivalent items for your own organization
1 Income from activities	1
2 Operating expenses	2
3 Staff costs	3
4 Bad debts	4
5 Depreciation and amortization	5
6 Operating profit (loss)	6
7 Profit (loss) before interest	7
8 Interest payable	8
9 Dividends payable	9
10 Retained profit (loss) for the year	10
11 Fixed assets	11
12 Stocks and work in progress	12
13 Debtors	13
14 Cash at bank and in hand	14
15 Net current assets (liabilities)	15
16 Creditors: amounts falling due after more than one year	16
17 Provisions for liabilities and charges	17
18 Total assets employed	18
19 Share capital	19
20 Revaluation reserve	20
21 Income and expenditure reserve	21
22 Other reserves	22
23 Total equity	23

Feedback

You may find some differences in terminology. However, for most of the items listed for Someplace Hospital you should find an equivalent for your own organization. Note that it is important that you are able to locate the relevant figures for the ratios you wish to use in the financial statements. The activities in this chapter will give you practice in doing so.

Throughout this series of activities the figures for Someplace Hospital will be in thousands of dollars. Those for your organization will relate to the currency in which your organization's accounts are stated. Make sure that you use the same order of magnitude for both numerator and denominator in the calculations so that, for example, if the numerator is stated in millions of dollars then the denominator is also stated in millions of dollars.

Financial position

The balance sheet reports the assets and liabilities of the company as at the date of the balance sheet. The ratios discussed here can be used to assess the financial health of the organization and, in particular, its ability to meet its short-term obligations. These ratios are also referred to as solvency ratios.

Working capital ratio

Also known as the current ratio, this compares the current assets with the current liabilities. You have seen in Chapter 13 how important it is to manage working capital. This ratio compares liabilities that are payable in the near future with cash and other short-term assets to determine the organization's ability to meet its obligations. The working capital ratio is simply current assets:current liabilities. This is simplified by dividing the current assets total by the current liabilities total:

$$\frac{\text{Current assets}}{\text{Current liabilities}}$$

It is then expressed in the form of a ratio x:1. You may also see this ratio expressed as x times. Textbooks sometimes recommend that the working capital ratio should be 2:1. However, this is rarely met in practice and the recommended ratio depends on the nature of the business but it is generally accepted that if the ratio is only around 1:1 this should be a cause for concern because there may not be sufficient assets to meet short-term obligations.

When looking at an organization's solvency it may also be helpful to compare the solvency ratios at different balance sheet dates. This may reveal a trend in solvency over the years. If the working capital ratio is steadily declining this may indicate a problem with working capital management. A sharp increase in solvency ratios may, on the other hand, suggest that there is cash lying idle.

Another way of looking at solvency ratios is to compare them with those for similar organizations.

Liquidity ratio

The *liquidity ratio* is also known as the *acid test ratio* because it is a more critical test of the organization's ability to meet its current liabilities than the working capital ratio.

This ratio excludes stock from the current assets on the grounds that it may not be possible to sell the stock in time to settle short-term liabilities. It is calculated as:

$$\frac{\text{Current assets} - \text{stock}}{\text{Current liabilities}}$$

Like the working capital ratio, the appropriate liquidity ratio is difficult to specify but it is nevertheless useful in highlighting any cause for concern in terms of the actual ratio, the trend in liquidity over the years or the level of liquidity of comparable organizations.

Gearing

While working capital and liquidity relate to the short-term solvency of an organization, *gearing* indicates whether an organization can meet its long-term liabilities. It is concerned with the way in which the ownership of the organization is structured. The term gearing, which may also be referred to as leverage, is used to describe the relationship between long-term finance, on which a fixed rate of interest is payable, and non-interest bearing finance such as reserves and shareholders' capital. The distinction is important because, with long-term liabilities there is a continuing obligation to meet interest payments. An organization that has a high proportion of interest-bearing debt may, in the long term, be unable to meet its finance charges.

Where organizations are funded by shareholders, companies with a large shareholding may have to distribute very much more in profits than in fixed interest. However, because the distribution of dividends is not compulsory while payment of interest is, companies in risky businesses where profit is not assured will be more likely to choose a low gearing ratio (i.e. more capital and less interest-bearing debt) than those in businesses where profit can be reliably anticipated. Given these trade-offs it is not usually possible to specify an ideal gearing ratio, although it is generally agreed that high gearing ratios carry a greater risk and should therefore be avoided.

Gearing ratios can be specified in a number of different ways according to the financing structure of the organization under review. For the purposes of this chapter a gearing ratio is defined as:

Interest-bearing finance:non-interest bearing finance

The gearing ratio can also be used as a basis for comparison of trends over a number of years or with the gearing of similar organizations.

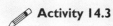 **Activity 14.3**

Now turn to the balance sheet of Someplace Hospital and that of your organization and complete the following tables, noting the implications of the ratios on a separate sheet of paper.

Table 14.2 Working capital ratios

	Year	Current assets	Current liabilities	Working capital ratio
Someplace Hospital	**2004**			
	2003			
Your organization				

Table 14.3 Liquidity (acid test) ratios

	Year	Current assets minus stock	Current liabilities	Liquidity ratio
Someplace Hospital	**2004**			
	2003			
Your organization				

Table 14.4 Gearing

	2004 $000	2003 $000
Someplace Hospital		
Interest-bearing debt		
Non-interest bearing funds:		
Share capital		
Revaluation reserve		
Income and Expenditure reserve		
Total non-interest bearing funds		
2004 gearing ratio		
2003 gearing ratio		
Your organization	**Year**	**Year**
Fixed interest funds		
Non-interest bearing funds:		
Total non-interest bearing funds		
2004 gearing ratio		
2003 gearing ratio		

When calculating the gearing ratio for Someplace Hospital, assume that all creditors falling due in more than one year are interest-bearing debt.

Feedback

Now compare the ratios you calculated for Someplace Hospital with those below.

Table 14.5 Working capital ratios (solution)

	Year	Current assets	Current liabilities	Working capital ratio
Someplace Hospital	**2004**	$22 565 000	$5 501 000	4.10:1
	2003	$12 404 000	$8 520 000	1.46:1

Someplace Hospital has a fairly high working capital ratio. This is significantly higher than at the last balance sheet date. However, the balance sheet shows that a very large part of the current assets is made up of debtors. If these could be converted into cash the organization may be in a position to invest its short-term funds. The balance sheet also reveals a substantial cash balance which has increased significantly from the (already high) cash balance at the beginning of the financial year. Could these assets be put to more productive use or invested where they would earn a good rate of interest?

Table 14.6 Liquidity ratios (solution)

	Year	Current assets minus stock	Current liabilities	Liquidity ratio
Someplace Hospital	**2004**	$21 800 000	$5 501 000	3.96:1
	2003	$11 778 000	$8 520 000	1.38:1

The stock figure makes very little difference here; the ratios are similar to the working capital ratios. A liquidity ratio of 1:1 (or near to that) would mean that the hospital could meet its short-term liabilities, so this suggests that the liquidity ratio is higher than it needs to be.

Table 14.7 Gearing (solution)

Someplace Hospital	2004 $000	2003 $000
Interest-bearing debt	7 798	0
Share capital:	11 220	11 220
Revaluation reserve	3 108	1 557
Income and Expenditure reserve	5 213	5 036
Total non-interest bearing funds	19 541	17 813
2004 gearing ratio: 0.40:1		
2003 gearing ratio – not applicable		

There was no interest-bearing debt on the balance sheet at 31 March 2003. The gearing has since risen to 0.40:1 indicating an increasing reliance on fixed interest funds. This is a significant change; as explained in Note 15 to the accounts, the hospital has taken a loan in order to build a new hospital wing.

Financial progress

The first item you are likely to look at on the income statement is the surplus for the year. However, on its own this is not a very informative figure. In the following activities you will learn about what performance ratios can tell you and how to apply them in practice.

There are many ways that the information in the income statement can be analysed; the choice of ratios will depend on your purpose. You may, for example, be focusing on income, in which case you may calculate:

• Percentage change in income between this year and last year which is calculated as follows:

$$\frac{\text{Change in this year's income}}{\text{Last year's income}} \times 100$$

• The percentage contribution of various activities/sources to total income (this information would be found in the notes to the accounts) and the change in contributions from one year to the next. While this is a relatively straight-forward exercise, it may be useful in highlighting any changes in the share of income from the different sources over a period of time.
• Operating profit/surplus as a percentage of income. In commercial organizations this is referred to as the *profit margin*, whereas in not-for-profit organizations it may be referred to as the *operating margin*. It is calculated as:

$$\frac{\text{Operating profit/surplus}}{\text{Income}} \times 100$$

If this ratio is deteriorating it could be because activity levels are lower because prices have been cut or the variable costs have gone up. Often it may be a combination of all three.

Other ratios focus on the ability of the organization to meet its interest and dividend commitments from the surplus it has generated:

• *Interest cover* calculates how many times the operating surplus generated during the year would cover the interest payable:

$$\frac{\text{Operating surplus}}{\text{Interest payable}}$$

• *Dividend cover* measures the proportion of the operating surplus that is distributed as dividends:

$$\frac{\text{Surplus after interest}}{\text{Dividends paid}}$$

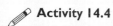 **Activity 14.4**

Now turn to the balance sheets of Someplace Hospital and of your organization and complete the following questions, noting the implications of the ratios you have calculated in each case.

1   What was the percentage change in income from continuing operations between the two years?

Table 14.8 Change in income

	Current year's income	Previous year's income	Difference	Previous year's income	Percentage change
Someplace Hospital					
Your organization					

2   Calculate the operating margins for both organizations.

Table 14.9 Operating margins

	Year	Operating profit/ surplus	Income from activities and continuing operations	Operating margin (%)
Someplace Hospital	2003/4			
	2002/3			
Your organization				

↻ **Feedback**

Check your findings for Someplace Hospital against those below. If you did not get them right then it will be worth checking your findings for your organization as well.

1   The percentage change in income is shown in Table 14.10.

Table 14.10 Change in income (solution)

	Current year's income	Previous year's income	Difference	Previous year's income	Percentage change
Someplace Hospital	$67 780 000	$59 687 000	$8 093 000	$59 687 000	13.56

In this case both income from activities and other operating income have been considered. However, for an organization such as Someplace Hospital which operates for profit, this information should be considered alongside information on the operating margins.

2   The operating margins are shown in Table 14.11.

Table 14.11 Operating margins (solution)

	Year	Operating profit/ surplus	Income from activities and continuing operations	Operating margin (%)
Someplace Hospital	2003/4	$1 011 000	$67 780 000	1.49
	2002/3	$1 229 000	$59 687 000	2.06

The operating margin for Someplace Hospital is relatively small and has fallen. Investors looking to maximize returns on their investment would be likely to question this. In public sector organizations that do not have a profit motive, operating margins are unlikely to be high and the use of any surplus is regulated by government (see the section on the residual claimant status in Chapter 1).

Combined ratios

There are a number of ratios that use information from both the income statement and the balance sheet in order to place performance in the context of the size of the organization (its assets and funding). These are referred to as combined ratios.

Return on capital employed

One of the most commonly used measures of operating performance is *return on capital employed (ROCE)*. This measure expresses the operating profit (i.e. the profit before interest and tax) as a percentage of the organization's relevant net assets and is calculated as follows:

$$\frac{\text{Profit/surplus on ordinary activities before interest and tax}}{\text{Capital employed}} \times 100$$

The definition of capital employed (which you may find referred to as 'relevant net assets') is the subject of much debate but it is generally agreed that it should include equity (described in Chapter 11 as the net assets of a company after all creditors have been paid off) or capital, and all sources of interest-bearing debt, both long and short term. To better reflect changes in capital employed during the year, average capital employed may be used. Average capital employed is calculated by adding the capital employed at the beginning and the end of the accounting period and dividing it by two.

This ratio is particularly useful because it can be used for comparison with alternative investments. It enables you to ask, 'If these funds (capital and long-term loans) had not been invested in this organization, what return might they have generated elsewhere (e.g. by comparing the return with the interest rates if the money was put in a bank account)?'

Asset utilization

Measures of asset utilization are an indication as to 'how hard the assets are working' by calculating how much income is being generated from each $1 invested in fixed assets. The higher the rate of asset turnover the greater the return on fixed asset investment. This is perhaps best used to determine the trend in asset turnover over a number of years. If the asset turnover is declining, it may be appropriate to review the need for the current level of assets. Might some be disposed of without an associated loss of income?

The definition of assets in this ratio is open to debate. Net assets, that is total assets less long- and short-term liabilities, is often favoured. However, others prefer to look only at fixed assets. Mellett *et al.* (1993) suggest that for a publicly-funded health system the *asset turnover ratio* should be calculated as:

$$\frac{\text{Income}}{\text{Average fixed assets}}$$

Activity 14.5

Using Someplace Hospital and your organization's accounts, complete the following.

1 Calculate the return on capital employed. Note that you will first need to calculate those assets that are relevant to this ratio. Use Table 14.12 to help you (you need not bother to calculate *average* capital employed – use the figure given as at the balance sheet dates). Figures have been supplied for Someplace Hospital where these are not included in the selected notes to the specimen accounts.

Table 14.12 Return on capital employed – Someplace Hospital

	2004 ($000)	2003 ($000)
Total capital and reserves		
Add: long-term creditors amounts falling due after one year		
Less: assets in the course of construction (see Note 11)		
Less: short-term investments (excluding cash at bank and in hand)	0	0
Plus: short-term loans	0	0
Plus: borrowed cash/overdrafts	0	0
Plus: finance lease creditors	0	0
Total		
Profit (loss) before interest and tax		
Return on capital – (profit before interest and tax divided by total) × 100		

Table 14.13 Return on capital employed – your organization

You may need to modify some of the headings in Column 1.

	Year ($000)	Year ($000)
Total capital and reserves		
Add: long-term creditors amounts falling due after one year		
Less: assets in the course of construction		
Less: cash invested (excluding cash at bank and in hand)		
Less: other reserves		
Plus: short-term loans		
Plus: borrowed cash/overdrafts		
Plus: finance lease creditors		
Total		
Profit (loss) or surplus (deficit) before interest and tax		
Return on capital – (profit/surplus before interest and tax divided by total) × 100		

2   Calculate the asset turnover. Note that you will first have to calculate average fixed assets by adding the figures for fixed assets at both balance sheet dates and dividing the total by two.

Table 14.14 Asset turnover

	Income from activities for 2003/4	Average fixed assets	Asset turnover
Someplace Hospital			
Your organization			

Feedback

1   The return on capital employed is shown in Table 14.15.

Table 14.15 Return on capital employed – Someplace Hospital (solution)

	2004 ($000)	2003 ($000)
Total capital and reserves	19 541	17 813
Add: long-term creditors amounts falling due after one year	7 798	0
Less: assets in the course of construction	(459)	(421)
Less: cash invested (excluding cash at bank and in hand)	0	0
Plus: short-term loans	0	0
Plus: borrowed cash/overdrafts	0	0
Plus: finance lease creditors	0	0
Total	26 880	17 392
Profit (loss) before interest and tax	868	1 195
Return on capital – (surplus divided by total) $\times$ 100	3.23%	6.87%

The return on capital employed has more than halved, falling from 6.87 per cent in 2002/3 to 3.23 per cent in 2003/4. But is this level of return good or bad? Your answer will depend on your reason for analysing the return. You may:

- wish to compare the return with that for previous years to see whether the return has risen or fallen; comparing actual surplus figures would not take into consideration any increase or decrease in capital employed in the way that the ratio does
- compare the return with that of other similar organizations

Don't overlook what may be obvious reasons for any change in the return on capital employed. In the case of Someplace Hospital, a substantial loan of almost $8 million has been taken out in the latest year to fund the building of a new wing. This downturn in the ROCE may need to be balanced against expectations of better returns when the building is operational.

Don't forget either that comparison with the return generated by commercial organizations or with commercial interest rates would not be valid for health care organizations that do not have an overriding profit motive.

2   Asset turnover is as follows.

Table 14.16 Asset turnover (solution)

	Income from activities for 2003/4 ($000)	Average fixed assets ($000)	Asset turnover
Someplace Hospital	62 417	(14 227 + 10 890) ÷ 2 = 12 559	4.97 times

It is not possible to compare this asset turnover with the previous year's activity because the opening balance for the previous year (2002) is not available. However, if your organization is comparable to Someplace Hospital, you may wish to compare the asset turnover ratios.

Working capital turnover ratios

You saw in Chapter 13 how important it is to exercise control over the various elements of working capital. Working capital ratios measure how long, on average, it takes to pay creditors, collect debts and use stocks, thus providing a useful monitoring tool. Average figures should be used; these are calculated by adding balances at the beginning and end of the accounting period and dividing them by two. In each case the ratio is multiplied by 365 so that it can be expressed in terms of days. These ratios are:

- $Creditor\ turnover = \dfrac{\text{average creditors}}{\text{purchases}} \times 365$

- $Debtor\ turnover = \dfrac{\text{average debtors}}{\text{income}} \times 365$

- $Stock\ turnover = \dfrac{\text{average stock}}{\text{stock consumption}} \times 365$

 Activity 14.6

How long, on average, do debtors take to settle their accounts with your organization?

Feedback

For Someplace Hospital the calculation of debtor turnover would be as follows:

$$\frac{(14{,}597{,}000 + 7{,}064{,}000) \div 2}{67{,}780{,}000} \times 365 = 58 \text{ days}$$

The level of debtors has risen significantly over the year, from $7,064,000 to $14,597,000 and the debtor turnover figure is 58 days which seems unacceptably high. In commercial organizations the normal time for settlement is 30 days from the date of statement. Statements are normally sent out on a monthly basis, so that debtors will, on average, have 15 days from the date of purchase (the invoice date) to the date the statement is issued, plus a further 30 days, making a total of 45 days to settle their accounts. However, your organization may have adopted a different payment code of practice, for example requiring organizations to pay all invoices within 30 days of receipt of goods or a valid invoice. This would reduce the average credit period to 30 days.

Limitations of financial ratios

It is important to remember that, although they can provide useful insights into organizational performance, financial ratios have several limitations:

- they are based on historical information and by the time they are used the organization's situation may be very different;
- they should only be used to compare similar organizations;
- there are a number of different definitions used in the calculation of several of the ratios, so it is important to make sure you are using the same definition when making comparisons;
- the balance sheet represents the financial position at a single point in time; this may not be representative of the situation throughout the financial year.

Key ratios at a glance

The following is a summary of the key ratios that you have used in this chapter.

Measuring financial position

Short-term solvency:

1 The working capital or current ratio = current assets/current liabilities.
2 The liquidity or acid test ratio = current assets − stock/current liabilities.

Long-term solvency:

3 Gearing ratio = interest-bearing funds/non-interest-bearing funds (or long-term liabilities/capital employed).

Measuring financial progress

Operating ratios:

1 Percentage income change: $\dfrac{\text{change in this year's income}}{\text{last year's income}} \times 100.$

2 Operating (profit) margin $= \dfrac{\text{operating surplus}}{\text{income}} \times 100.$

Investment ratios. These measure the ability to pay returns on sums invested in the organization:

3   Interest cover = operating surplus/interest charge.
4   Dividend cover = surplus after interest/dividend.

Combined ratios

These use information from income statement and balance sheet:

1   Asset turnover = income/average fixed assets.
2   ROCE = surplus on ordinary activities before interest × 100/capital employed.
3   Working capital turnover rates:

   a) creditor turnover = average creditors × 365/purchasers
   b) debtor turnover = average debtors × 365/income
   c) stock turnover = average stock × 365/consumption of supplies.

Activity 14.7 is designed to test your understanding of ratios and their uses.

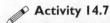

Activity 14.7

1   Your board is considering an investment of $3,000,000 which is to be financed by a bank loan. What ratios are the bankers likely to look at when considering your application?

2   You consider entering an agreement with a supplier which involves a regular order of consumables worth $10,000 per month. As you are a new customer the supplier requires your latest published financial account to obtain some information about your financial position. What information is the supplier likely to look at?

3   Explain what is meant by a high-geared organization as compared to a low-geared one.

4   You are supervising a health care organization which has increased its operating margin from 10 to 15 per cent. What issues would you consider?

5   You received an audit report on a health centre that is financed by several insurance companies which are billed for their patients. The acid test ratio was 0.6 and the debtor turnover was 50 days. What should management do?

6   An accountant has supplied you with a set of ratios which have been extracted from last year's financial accounts of a health care organization which is considered for a merger. Do ratios and the financial statements tell you enough about the organization's performance?

Feedback

1 Gearing and interest cover. The gearing ratio is a measure of financial risk that measures the proportion of debt (the long-term liabilities) to the capital employed. The interest cover gives account of the organization's ability to service an extra debt.

2 The supplier would be interested in your short-term solvency. As they want to minimize the risk of failing to get your money they will look at your liquidity by assessing the cash flow statement and calculating the current and the acid test ratio. However, these ratios have limits as your liquidity may have changed during the current financial year.

3 Gearing measures the capital structure. A high-geared organization would have a dangerously high interest burden while a low-geared organization has a better ratio of capital to debt.

4 The operating margin indicates the operating surplus as a proportion of income. While a business company with a high profit margin (the equivalent to the operating margin) would be considered successful, this may be different in public sector organizations. You would look at the sources of the surplus and assess whether the prices were set too high or the surplus was achieved by cutting corners resulting in a quality decline. Most countries regulate the profits of public sector organizations by setting cut-off points or by fiscal collection of the operating surplus.

5 The organization could improve its liquidity (which is low as indicated by the liquidity rate) by improving debt collection. As a rule the debts should be collected as quickly as possible to have enough liquid funds for paying creditors.

6 Clearly not. Isolated account information can be virtually useless. Ratios are always the starting point of an investigation rather than the answer. They need to be considered in context, over time, compared to the average performance of similar organizations. To validate accounting information you need to look at other issues, such as human resource implications, industrial relations, the extent of competition and future health policy plans. You may also need more detailed financial information such as achievement against budgets or contracts, a breakdown of cost per department/patient/activity/staff member. What makes financial accounts and ratios valuable is their *context*.

Summary

Performance ratios provide the basis for comparison of information contained in the financial statements either on a year-to-year basis or with similar organizations. Balance sheet ratios are mainly concerned with the standing of the organization and focus on working capital, liquidity and gearing. Performance ratios focus on the income statement and on profitability, while combined ratios include such indicators of activity as asset turnover and working capital turnover ratios.

Perhaps the most commonly used ratio is the return on capital employed, which states the operating surplus as a percentage of the relevant net assets employed (or capital employed) in the organization.

Reference

Mellett, H., Marriott, N. and Harries, S. (1993) *Financial Management in the NHS: A Manager's Handbook*. London: Chapman & Hall.

SECTION 4

Financial control and information systems

15 Financial and management reporting

Overview

This is the first of six chapters on financial control and information systems. Information produced by an accounting system must be accurate, timely and relevant. It is important that the accounting system is designed to meet not only the statutory requirements for the production of financial accounting statements but also the internal information needs of the organization. Accounting systems must also be secure; there is a duty on managers in both the public and private sectors to ensure the safe handling of the assets belonging to the organization. Where cash is concerned this presents a particular responsibility, especially where large sums are involved. It is important, therefore, that they have in place a system of financial controls designed to prevent fraud or theft. Public sector organizations are also subject to a number of regulations that ensure they meet the objectives set out for them. Chapters 15 to 17 cover accounting systems, their control and the external regulations imposed on organizations.

In Chapters 18 and 19 the focus is on information, with a discussion of information systems to meet the changing information needs in health systems and of the investment appraisal techniques that can provide the necessary information when making capital investment decisions. Finally, Chapter 20 introduces financial aspects of project management.

The financial and management reporting systems in your organization provide the information on which you judge your performance and on which your performance is judged. It is important for you to know how these systems work because when investigating performance you need to know where in the system to look to confirm what is going on. Often you will find that a hitch or error in the data entered in the system causes an apparent problem. It will save you a lot of time if you can investigate and resolve this speedily instead of performing complex calculations to justify data that are really just an accounting error or, worse perhaps, to accept responsibility for something that shouldn't even be there. This chapter will give you the skills to find your way round your financial and management reporting systems and even participate in a more informed way in formulating proposals for new systems by combining health care insights with knowledge of reporting systems to ensure you get the system that meets your needs.

Learning objectives

By the end of this chapter you should be able to:

- explain the flow of information in a financial reporting system
- explain the flow of information in a management reporting system
- explain the purpose of a case-mix management system
- describe the financial and management reporting systems for your organization

Key terms

Audit trail A tool for checking data integrity, allowing each transaction to be tracked down from the highest level of aggregation to the single entry of the feeder system and vice versa.

Budget summarization hierarchy A budget structure reflecting the distribution of financial responsibility and accountability within large organizations. Single budget items of sub-units are combined to become totals of the next level in the hierarchy.

Case-mix system An information system combining patient-related activity data with financial data on resource use.

Feeder system The data input system of the financial reporting system responsible for the recording and processing of all financial transactions.

Financial reporting system An information system performing all aspects of the accounting process, involving the recording and processing of financial transactions as well as the producing of reports for various purposes.

General ledger (nominal ledger) The main account book which consolidates the record of financial activities and allows the bottom line of net earnings to be calculated.

Management reporting system The information system supporting the running of an organization. Management reports include both financial and non-financial information and can be produced for either strategic or operational purposes.

Financial and management reporting systems

Managers have to rely on accurate, timely and relevant information to be able to make decisions. Information management is a fundamental activity to facilitate communication within the organization and with external customers. This key function of running any organization is supported by financial and management *information systems*. These systems assist in coping with the large quantities of data that are produced on a daily basis in the organization. Typically, this involves condensing and fusing large amounts of data from different sources, such as financial, patient and activity records, into a manageable number of key variables, which provide aggregated information for an understanding of the present conditions and making decisions on the future of the organization. The basic process underlying information systems can be described by a simple input/output model: data → information → message.

- Data are the input of the communication process. They are numbers or symbols which need an interpretative context to allow their significance to be analysed. So you need some auxiliary information to make sense of data.
- Information is a translation of data with sufficient context added to enable them to be analysed and evaluated.
- The message (output) is an interpretative statement derived from information. Messages make sense of the information and convey a meaning. They pursue distinct objectives and are tailored to the need of their users.

Figure 15.1 illustrates how this process might look in monitoring the performance of a health care organization. Inputs capture a range of data sources such as activity, patient, financial and market-related data. These are analysed and used in specific contexts, such as measuring service quality, financial performance or organizational growth. The output is presented in the form of ideas, reports and analyses which are distributed according to the organization's communication strategy. Reports and analyses are produced:

- *periodically*, for example, on a monthly or quarterly basis or annually like financial accounts;
- *at trigger points*, for example, when a loss is expected or reserves are being consumed, or clinical activity deviates from the planned level or at any other financial warning point;
- *on request*, for example, for specific projects or for assessing returns on a new investment.

These different types of report are usually produced by the finance department though large health care organizations may use dedicated professional staff who integrate financial and clinical information and report to the top management. Under a policy of financial transparency and accountability, unit managers and clinical staff are also involved in producing and using reports according to their individual level of responsibility.

Good management reports rarely present long tables with hundreds of figures; rather they are short and clear to make the message easily understood. While detailed numbers are important for bookkeepers and accountants, decision-makers

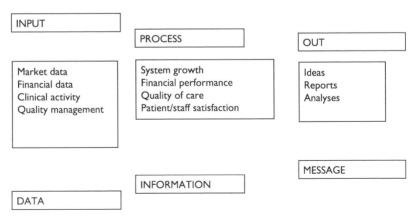

Figure 15.1 System for monitoring the performance of a health care organization

need knowledge of the order of magnitude, the key relationships and trends of financial processes. In presenting financial information, written, orally or on-screen, meaningful diagrams and charts can say more than a thousand words and tables with rounded figures (in most cases only the two first digits matter, for example, 1.5 million instead of 1,545,645) should be used (Allen and Myddleton 1992). Generally, when producing a report the following criteria should be met:

- *relevance:* reports should avoid presenting irrelevant materials and focus on the key information for decision-making;
- *user-orientation:* reports should be tailored to the needs of the audience who may not all be financial experts;
- *balance and trueness:* the information should not be distorted in aggregating the data and the report should not over-simplify complex issues; alternative options for decision-making should be clearly presented;
- *continuity:* to allow financial performance to be compared over time, definitions of the items reported should not change;
- *timeliness:* reports should provide the most up-to-date information in order to support rational decision-making;
- *efficiency:* limits in time and costs of producing reports have to be observed. The costs of producing the information should be justified by the benefits provided.

Financial reporting systems

You should note that the term 'information system' does not necessarily mean that IT is used. It could be a simple manual bookkeeping system or manual records of clinical activity. The traditional model of a financial reporting system is centred on the *general ledger* (or main account book) which consolidates the record of financial activities and allows the bottom line of net earnings to be calculated. However, increasingly IT-based reporting systems are used; these can cope more easily with large numbers of financial transactions and provide a range of automated report-producing facilities for internal and external users. Automated reporting extends to both management and financial reports and includes a range of tools for budget planning and control as well as treasury and asset management. Output can be displayed in various ways such as the general ledger, accounts receivable, accounts payable and the corresponding sub-ledger accounts. The actual recording of the data, the many financial transactions, is processed in *feeder systems*, which provide data input for the financial reporting system.

A large organization has many different feeder systems which include for example:

- salaries and wages;
- creditor payments;
- stock;
- debtors;
- capital charges;
- travel expenses;
- other expenses and so on.

Each feeder system is designed to record the financial transactions related to a specific area. The feeder system for the payroll records all kind of payments to staff, the creditor feeder system ensures that all invoices received are included in the accounts, and so on.

Because the data are aggregated to higher levels in the ledger system it is important that the integrity of the information is maintained. This can be checked by the *audit trail* by which each piece of information can be tracked down from the highest level of aggregation to the single entry of the feeder system and vice versa. Each position is assigned a unique identifier, the financial code, to enable verification of the integrity of data. For example, the overall monthly expenditure for nurses as it appears in the general ledger can be traced back by use of the coding system to Nurse A, B, C and so on. An intact audit trail is a key requirement of financial control which is mandatory for the detection of unexplained losses, suspected fraud, possible data entry errors or any other inconsistency that might arise from the financial report.

Apart from being able to audit the information, another important requirement is that the data are correctly entered and up to date. Many of the inputs need to be updated on a weekly or even daily basis in order to obtain timely financial reports; incorrect coding could largely reduce the value of the reports. According to Mellet *et al.* (1993) the most common types of error include:

- missing codes, i.e. a transaction has been processed without any code being attached;
- invalid codes, i.e. codes have been entered that do not exist in the financial reporting system;
- incorrect valid codes, i.e. the codes exist, but are incorrect for the particular transaction.

Thus a basic knowledge of the most common errors that might occur is helpful when analysing the consistency of your accounts.

Activity 15.1

It is important to identify the feeder systems because the data are incorporated in the reports on which performance is judged and decisions taken. To be in a position to investigate and justify the performance for which you have budgetary responsibility you need to know where the data come from.

1 Describe the key inputs and outputs of the financial reporting system used in your organization. In Table 15.1 list the feeder systems and the data these contain.
2 Find out how the audit trail works in the financial reports that are available to you. For what purpose is it used?

Table 15.1 Inputs into the financial reporting system

Feeder system	Description of the data processed
(Example) Salaries and wages	SSI System weekly payroll for manual operatives grades c–e and h–i

Feedback

1 You should be able to identify all the feeder systems that impact on the management reports and your own budget. Remember to include both computerized and manual systems, since both of these potentially impact on the reporting systems.

2 An audit trail enables information produced by the system to be traced back to the originating entries and documentation. In a manual accounting system it could be a number code that is attached to each transaction. In computerized systems the audit trail is usually created by an electronic log of every transaction. The audit trail is used for internal management control purposes, so that managers can obtain further information on any item they wish to investigate. It is also used by both internal and external auditors to satisfy them that the system is operating as it should.

Management reporting systems

Management reporting refers to a wide range of considerations related to running an organization. The nature of the reports can vary according to the purpose for which they are produced and may include both financial and non-financial information. As shown in Figure 15.2 a basic distinction can be made between management reports for strategic and for operational purposes.

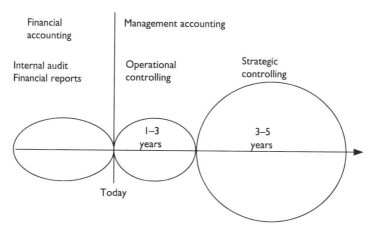

Figure 15.2 Time frame and purposes of financial and management accounting

Strategic reporting

Strategic reports assist in securing the financial stability of the organization in the long run and serve a range of purposes:

1 *Planning:* examples include business plans for new projects which require income and expenditure to be projected over several years. At a larger scale donor consortia and government may develop sector-wide plans for health care

expenditure over three or five years. Other strategic issues requiring accurate financial information are related to mergers or acquisitions of new facilities, or finding strategic partners for service expansion.

2 *Market analyses:* these help managers to assess the strengths and weaknesses of the organization's own position and examine the critical external factors that impinge on the performance of the organization. In addition to financial input these reports combine information from different data sources, for example on provider density, socioeconomic data on the population served, nature and volume of the services provided in a region and development of the insurance market for health insurance.

3 *Customer relations:* an important aim of strategic management reporting is to assist in the development of long-term customer relations, for example, with referring institutions, patient organizations, primary care doctors and medical suppliers. A hospital would also assess patient satisfaction and set targets for improvement on a regular basis.

4 *Evaluation:* management reports are also produced for evaluation of new approaches to service delivery and to financing of services or the introduction of new provider payment methods. For example, introducing performance-related pay in a health centre requires careful attention to the effects on volume and quality of the services provided and of the transaction costs involved. Management investigations and financial reports produced may convince purchasers of the new method of service delivery and are fundamental in calculating prices for services and gaining new contracts.

Operational reporting

Operational reporting is helpful in securing the quality and efficiency of service provision in the short run. Reports are produced for a range of purposes such as ensuring that costs are controlled, liquidity is maintained and agreed returns are achieved. The aim is to establish an early warning system that allows the financial risk of the organization to be assessed quickly. The key approach is *variance analysis* – the comparison of planned and actual data of a range of measures such as asset adequacy, liquidity, operative performance and activity data such as occupancy or numbers of cases treated.

In an environment which uses devolved budgets, unit managers may receive a monthly or quarterly budget performance report allowing them to compare planned and actual expenditure (as seen in Chapter 7). A particular focus may be directed on critical areas, for which separate reports may be produced. Staff budgets provide information on the planned and actual whole time equivalent (WTE) staff numbers, including information on turnover and absenteeism to be able to react quickly in filling gaps and deploying staff efficiently. Drug budgets inform on actual and planned level of expenditure for medicines on each individual patient to monitor rationality of prescribing.

A typical budget hierarchy reflecting the divisional structure of a government health system is shown in Figure 15.3. Note that the single budget items of the sub-units are combined to become totals of the next level in the hierarchy. The degree of accountability and discretion given to influence costs may vary largely. But even where unit managers are granted fewer powers in influencing performance, targets may be agreed for particular areas, such as for drug expenditure, or at least feedback

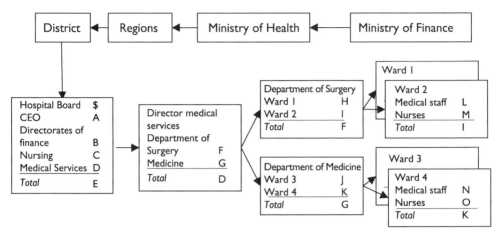

Figure 15.3 Budget hierarchy in a public health system

Source: Adapted from Mellet *et al.* (1993)

containing financial information is given to clinical staff in order to improve behaviour in resource use.

It is important to be aware that devolved budgets are of limited effect if the top level restricts the powers of unit managers in decision-making in key areas of cost control, for example in employment decisions or choice of suppliers. Unit managers can only be held responsible for those aspects they can significantly influence. Thus the reasons for poor performance should be carefully analysed before taking action and it should be considered that budget variances could have many different causes, internal and external to the organization. Obviously mismanagement and inappropriate provider behaviour are important internal ones. New technology such as new drugs or new procedures should be assessed carefully before being introduced into clinical practice. However, there are a range of external factors that are more difficult or even impossible to control such as financial risks linked to changes in:

- morbidity, for example an epidemic outbreak or new diseases;
- consumer demand, for example service use may change due to unforeseen increase in travel costs, changes in preferences for specific treatments or the opening of new facilities by competing providers;
- regulations, for example, government may change price regulation for drugs or impose new rules for investments or staff working hours;
- inflation and currency exchange rates – the effects of the former are particularly difficult to plan in countries with hyperinflation, likewise volatile exchange rates may affect costs of imported goods and services in an unforeseeable way.

In recent years efforts have been made to contain risks arising from provider behaviour, particularly from inappropriate clinical decisions that can have a huge impact on costs. Therefore management reports increasingly integrate clinical data to ensure that the most efficient ways of treating patients are used. To reduce variance in clinical decision-making and achieve value for money, various approaches have been employed such as:

- applying clinical guidelines based on cost-effective pathways of care;
- utilization review, employed to assess the appropriateness of the services provided, for example, of hospital treatment, before or after admission;
- peer review, assessing the appropriateness of clinical decisions;
- quality circles as a means of agreeing on the best way of organizing and delivering care.

All of these approaches aim to optimize resource use and may use internal and external data for comparing performance.

Activity 15.2

The more devolved the budgeting system, the more levels there will be in the budget hierarchy. Knowing where your budget is located in a structure like this is very helpful because it indicates to you:

- where and how your financial performance is reported upwards to top management
- the subsidiary management reports to examine and check before reviewing the source data from the feeder systems

Draw a budget hierarchy for your own organization, showing how it fits into the health system in your country. If you are unable to identify the hierarchy, ask members of your finance department if they can describe it to you.

Feedback

Budget summarization hierarchies vary for different organizations depending on the degree to which their budget systems are devolved. However, these should show a clear series of pathways between the top summary or master budget and the subsidiary budgets that support this by providing progressively more detailed and specialized information. Even if you don't have devolved budgets in your organization, think of its larger context and identify where the money comes from. A typical pathway involves the Ministry of Finance, the Ministry of Health, regions, districts and facilities as shown in Figure 15.3.

Case-mix management

A traditional and eternal management problem that besets all organizations is how to link activities and costs. The idea of a case-mix management system is to help management to relate patient information to workload data, and details of resources consumed. Case-mix models are part of the hospital information system but they are also increasingly used in ambulatory care. As a hospital manager who is concerned with service planning you need to answer questions such as:

- If a service is expanded by a certain amount, how many extra beds and theatre sessions will be required?
- What will it cost?

These information systems combine patient activity with information on resource consumption in the form of financial data. The key problem is that average costs are not responsive to projected activity changes, so a marginal approach needs to be used instead.

1 Some models are based on cost triggers, which record changes in numbers of patient days per speciality, opening or closing a ward, changing the number of operating sessions etc. to calculate the cost of a given case-mix.
2 Others record activity for each patient and calculate costs per episode, which are then grouped to analyse total cost or cost per case. Their common element is a patient classification system that allows relating the type of patients treated to resource use.

One of the most common systems are diagnosis-related groups (DRGs), which were developed at Yale University in the 1980s and were first used in reimbursing treatment of Medicare patients in the USA (Fetter *et al.* 1980). Since then the system has been refined and adapted to different uses and settings. DRGs are now used in hospital management in many low-income countries. A range of middle-income countries have also experimented and gained experience with case-mix systems. For managers the main function of DRGs is to provide the basis for prospective case-based payment of hospital services, though case-mix systems are being used for a range of other purposes such as:

• *Research:* DRGs provide information on service use and allow comparisons of geographical areas.
• *Planning:* a number of countries use case-mix systems for strategic planning and contracting for the hospital sector. In population level models, case-mix information is used to simulate costs and consequences of changes in service provision, for example the move to an essential package of health care which comprises a range of defined high-priority preventive and curative interventions that maximize health gains.
• *Resource allocation:* case-mix systems are used in a number of countries to allocate and devolve budgets. Because the approach relies on objective data it is less prone to political influences.
• *Quality management:* DRGs assist in clinical audit and quality assurance. They can be used to develop clinical pathways and guidelines, and provide information to compare the performance of health care organizations across a wide range of resource measures.

Typically a DRG system used for financial management combines information from the following sources:

• *patient data* (demographic and clinical, such as age, sex, diagnosis, comorbidity and complications);
• *activity data* (on types of procedure and interventions received, length of stay);
• *financial data* (cost profiles per individual case or agreed cost weights).

Each case is assigned the appropriate diagnostic and procedural category and here again the quality of coding is paramount. For example, in the Australian DRG system the code consists of three distinct elements which reveal:

• the main diagnostic category is based on the International Classification of Diseases, tenth revision (ICD10);

- the type of treatment received;
- the level of resource use, based on an index measuring clinical complexity and comorbidity of the case.

Thus in the code B70A (for stroke with severe complications), the letter B refers to the main diagnosis and signifies that the DRG belongs to the broad category of disorders of the nervous system, the figure 70 specifies in detail the diagnosis/procedure, for example, stroke with medical treatment, and the letter A signifies the highest level of resource use out of four categories A–D.

Table 15.2 shows an example of four DRGs of a stroke unit, reflecting different reimbursement levels according to case complexity and resource use.

Table 15.2 Four adjacent DRGs of a stroke unit

DRG	Text	Number of cases	Cost weight	Average length of stay (d)	Reimbursement per case ($)
B70A	Stroke with catastrophic complications/ comorbidity	10	1.78	10.7	2670
B70B	Stroke with severe complications/ comorbidity	25	1.389	11.5	2084
B70C	Stroke without severe or catastrophic complication	35	1.169	9.8	1754
B70D	Stroke, patient died within four days of admission	2	0.654	2.4	981

As you can see it is particularly important to capture the correct level of clinical complexity since much of the hospital income may depend on correct coding. Increasingly this job is done by specifically skilled coders who review medical records for the assignment of the correct DRG. Where several thousand cases have to be processed, coding is supported by an analytical software tool, a so-called 'grouper'.

 Activity 15.3

As you have seen, case-mix models can be used for service planning as well as for financial planning. If a case-mix management system is used by your organization, list the information on which it is based. Alternatively, if you do not have a case-mix management system, think how you would design one, listing the information that would be needed.

Feedback

In either case, your answer should be structured under three headings:

1 Financial information needed for the case-mix management system.

2 Patient information needed for the case-mix management system.

3 Activity information needed for the case-mix management system.

The integration of financial and management information

Increasingly, IT systems are used to integrate financial and management reporting. An integrated system will support all kinds of automated analyses and reports for internal and external purposes. The centrepiece of such a system is the financial accounting system. Connected with this are a range of modules which serve decision-making in the areas of:

- *Customer relations:* special modules help coordinate patient care from pre-admission to discharge, assuring continuity of care. They provide facilities such as billing, creditor management and communication with providers, patients, external physicians, employees, donors and other key stakeholders.
- *Human resources:* a module integrating payroll functions with the personnel information system to enable planning and managing of staff efficiently.
- *Logistics:* applications supporting the procurement and inventory functions for drugs and other consumables and other activities such as ordering, purchasing, stock management, maintenance and facility management.
- *Quality management:* supporting functions for internal and external clinical audit, accreditation and quality planning.

Bridging the digital divide between low- and high-income countries is a key concern for international development. While low-income countries use IT increasingly for central financial planning and budget control, it is used less frequently inpatient care, due to the high costs involved and lack of IT skills. Yet in some areas efforts have been made to provide IT support for processing data about health status, scheduling visits for immunization, and maternal and child health programmes as well as various outreach services. Thereby, handwritten reports are replaced and health data gathered in primary care are communicated to the district and regional levels for strategic planning and decision-making (Sastry 2003).

Summary

Information systems can cope with large quantities of data and are designed to support managers in internal and external communication. Every financial transaction needs to be recorded at the earliest possible point and in such a way as to support both statutory financial reporting requirements and management reporting requirements. Raw data are initially entered into feeder systems and transactions are then entered (usually in batches or automatically transferred) into the main ledger systems which should be designed in such a way as to facilitate the production of annual accounts to meet statutory requirements, budget reports and various other management reports as and when they are called for. An audit trail enables you to trace information produced back to the original source documents that gave rise to the accounting entries. Budget summaries show a clear series of pathways between the top summary or master budget and the subsidiary budgets that support this by providing progressively more detailed and more specialized information. Case-mix management involves the matching of patient activity or workload information to the relevant resource consumption information in an attempt to link activities and costs.

References

Allen, M.W. and Myddleton, D.R. (1992) *Essential Management Accounting*. London: Prentice-Hall Europe.

Fetter, R., Shin, Y., Freeman, J., Averill, R. and Thompson, J. (1980) Case-mix definition by diagnosis-related groups, *Medical Care*, 18(2): 1–53.

Mellett, H., Marriott, N. and Harries, S. (1993) *Financial Management in the NHS: A Manager's Handbook*. London: Chapman & Hall.

Sastry, C.L.R. (2003) The India Health Care Project: information technology in developing countries, *IFIP Newsletter*, 13:1.

16 Financial control

Overview

Financial controls are necessary to ensure that opportunities for mismanagement, fraud and corruption do not exist or are kept to an absolute minimum. Managers are charged with responsibility for safeguarding the assets of an organization and must actively ensure that appropriate controls are in place. In this chapter you will first learn about the need for financial control and then go on to examine an example that will help develop your awareness of the need for financial controls along with your ability to review control systems already in place.

Learning objectives

By the end of this chapter you should be able to:

- discuss the need for internal financial controls
- describe the various financial control systems operating in your organization
- review the effectiveness of the control systems, making recommendations for improvements where necessary

Key terms

Corruption Misuse of a position for dishonest gain, particularly the offering, giving, soliciting or acceptance of an inducement or reward, which may influence the action of the position-holder.

Financial controls Systems to maintain probity at all levels of the organization through adherence to rules of governance, laws, financial regulations and internal policies.

Fraud An intentional deception or misrepresentation that could result in some unfair gain. Financial fraud may involve activities such as forgery, falsification or alteration of documents as well as theft, destruction or misappropriation of funds, or misuse of facilities.

High-level controls Actions implemented at board level and above, as part of the governance system, to ensure that budgetary controls and audit systems are in place.

Low-level controls Actions specific to operational aspects of the organization, for example separating duties to minimize the risk of fraud in recording and authorizing of financial transactions.

Mismanagement, fraud and corruption

In recent years several cases of fraud and mismanagement have rocked the financial sectors around the world. High-profile cases such as Enron and WorldCom have not, however, been restricted to the private sector. You have only to think of the European Commission being unable to account for many billions of expenditure or the Eurostats scandal which revealed a total lack of audit trail that enabled officials to divert millions of euros into secret bank accounts. Or think of reports of $3 million siphoned out of Kenya through corrupt deals under the former government.

The discovery of such cases gives rise to the speculation as to how much fraud and corruption is actually discovered, and of that which is discovered, how much is reported publicly.

In health services corruption and fraud cannot be neglected. For example, the British NHS employs more than 400 local specialists to fight prescription fraud and the unit has reduced the annual damage caused by fraud and corruption from £117 million to £47 million within four years (*Guardian*, 18 February 2004).

- *Corruption* is the offering, giving, soliciting or acceptance of an inducement or reward, which may influence the action of any person.
- *Fraud* is the intentional distortion of financial statements or other records by persons internal or external to the organization which is carried out to conceal the misappropriation of assets for gain.

Corruption in the health sector

Corruption is a worldwide concern, so you should spend a little time considering the different forms in the health sector and what could contribute to eradicating these practices or at least limiting their impact. More generally, corruption is 'the misuse of power entrusted to a person for personal gain' (Transparency International 2004). A distinction can be made between corruption 'according to rule' where preferential treatment is expected for something the bribe receiver is required to do anyway, for example to give a patient access to a treatment they are entitled to receive, corruption 'against the rule' which expects the bribe receiver to do something unlawful, for example to participate in a fraud.

Although many countries and international organizations have made progress in fighting fraud and bribery, there are large international differences in culture, corporate governance and the prevalence and acceptability of these practices. The various forms of corruption extend from political corruption and vote-buying through corrupt business practices of large organizations to dishonest behaviour of staff who deliver services. High corruption levels are frequently related to shortcomings in the legal system, perverse economic incentives and lack of regulatory frameworks. Corruption is less likely to be supported where clear, accurate and formal rules of governance are accepted and enforced.

Corruption in the health sector has many different faces and involves different settings, for example at the interface between:

- *Private and public sector:* where bribing of public officials to gain contracts is not uncommon. A particularly vulnerable area is the procurement and distribution of medical supplies. As a large number of people (in public administration, donor agencies, procurement offices, pharmacies and health care organizations) are involved in distribution between manufacturer and patient, corruption can occur at any stage of this process. Fraudulent practices include bribery, kickbacks or rebates as well as excessive pricing of articles and sharing profits between the supply company and the public official. Stock in hospitals and public pharmacies may be pilfered and resold on the black market.
- *The medical-industrial complex and health professionals:* institutionalized corruption occurs in the form of travel scholarships, sponsored meetings and rebates granted by the industry. Corruption of the medical literature has occurred where authors have failed to disclose their conflict of interest and are paid by industry to produce results in favour of their products (such as tobacco and pharmaceuticals). Open and disguised forms of bribing to influence prescribing behaviour and other extreme forms of unethical conduct of the pharmaceutical industry have received much attention in recent years. Many countries and professional associations have enacted codes of conduct regulating contacts between physicians and the industry.
- *Staff and patients:* unofficial user fees are common in many countries where incentives to produce a service are lacking or health professionals are poorly paid. In many transitional countries of Central and Eastern Europe, 'under the table money' is still common as part of the doctor's fee. Sometimes it is difficult to draw a line between a culturally accepted custom and corruption. While in some countries gifts are considered as a friendly gesture to thank medical staff for their services, in other countries bribing is indispensable to get access to care, shorten waiting times or receive a better quality of treatment.
- *Providers, patients and third-party payers:* corruption can be linked with various forms of health care, for example, submitting false claims to insurance companies or government, who may be billed excessively or billed for services not rendered. In principle all people entitled to make payment claims can be involved in this kind of fraud, doctors as well as patients, pharmacies and drug companies. Claims have been submitted for dead patients, for fake prescriptions or 'ghost' delivery of drugs to health centres or distribution of expired drugs.
- *Donors and recipients of external aid:* in external aid, donors and recipient governments have increased their efforts to protect funds from corruption. However, donor countries can be part of the problem and particularly those which do not penalize bribing of foreign officials have been urged to change their anti-corruption laws. In low-income countries corruption is not only a governance problem but also a development problem, which is intertwined with inefficiencies in services, low public sector pay and lack of accountability. Capacity-building and institutional strengthening are key in improving financial controls and procurement systems. At the societal level, building coalitions with stakeholders and involving civil society groups is fundamental to increasing the transparency of political and economic processes and to prevent corruption at the higher levels of the political hierarchy (OECD 2003).

Activity 16.1

Think of examples of corruption and fraud that have occurred recently in the health sector of your country. What are the potential consequences of these practices for the organizations involved and the health system in general?

 Feedback

Though norms and values vary between countries, you will be able to provide an account specific to your country. All these forms of corruption impinge on performance since they affect the credibility of the organization and involve additional cost to the user. Of course, there is a range of views on corruption and a range of cultural differences in the acceptance of these practices. Sometimes corruption is seen as just oiling the wheels, or in economic terms, as enhancing efficiency by giving officials an incentive to work (Weiner 1962). However, in real terms the costs of corruption add substantially to the costs of health care which the individual and society have to bear. At service delivery level these effects may become visible in supply shortages, deprivation of facilities or waste of resources as funds are channelled from patients with clinical needs to those able to pay. At systems level, corruption distorts competition and creates a climate of distrust and indifference which may deter donors or investors from working with the organizations involved. Corrupt managers cause frustration and demotivation among staff, thereby undermining the reputation and accountability of the organization.

Preventing fraud

As you have seen, health care fraud is a potential threat to the efficient functioning of the health system, which is often (but not necessarily) related to corruption. Fraudulent behaviour includes a range of activities such as forgery, falsification or alteration of documents as well as theft, destruction or misappropriation of funds, or misuse of facilities for personal gain. Normally any organization has policies describing the responsibilities of staff and managers in preventing and detecting fraud and of the procedures for taking disciplinary and legal action. Any member of staff should feel responsible for safeguarding the resources in their area of responsibility and feel encouraged to report any irregularity to their superiors. Managers should be aware of the potential misdemeanours in their area and ensure that adequate controls are in place. They are responsible for enforcing the organization's policies and procedures, including the protection of staff who make public their concerns (whistleblowers) from reprisal.

IT fraud

The increasing use of IT and the growth of complex information management systems have resulted in increased opportunities for deception and such behaviour can lose organizations a great deal of money either through fraud or through system breakdowns. Therefore, organizations need to actively promote policies and control systems to prevent:

- computer fraud in the form of unauthorized alteration of data, programs or output;
- theft of data or software and the illegal use of software;
- hacking (gaining unauthorized access to a computer system) and sabotaging the computer process by causing damage to the system;
- viruses, worms and trojans, or other unknowingly distributed programs designed to corrupt the computer process.

Despite the increasing significance of external violations, IT systems have been found to be more vulnerable to violations committed by internal staff. Of 114 cases of IT fraud the majority were committed by managers (45 per cent) and by clerical staff (32 per cent). Only 13 per cent of the cases were committed by external intruders. Most of the cases occurred in purchase and payment. Common reasons were inadequate separation of duties, false documentation, inadequate controls, collusion, negligence, lack of internal review and improper authorization (Calderon and Green 1994).

To prevent IT fraud it is recommended that organizations undertake the following measures.

1   Carry out a detailed and comprehensive risk analysis to identify those areas of the system that are open to fraud and abuse.
2   Introduce a computer security strategy across the organization. Such a strategy will define access levels to the system for different personnel so that unauthorized staff do not have access to sensitive or vulnerable information.
3   Promote staff awareness of the need for IT security and the possible risks of IT fraud.
4   Carry out a regular programme of computer audit intended to detect any possible IT fraud.

 Activity 16.2

Make enquiries into the measures in your organization designed to ensure the security of information systems. Note that 'information systems' means not only financial information systems but also patient records and administration systems. The organization does not have to have a sophisticated computer-based system before security measures are necessary – this issue is relevant to all organizations.

 Feedback

You may have found that a range of policies, standards and procedures for information security are applied in your organization. Quite often a senior member of staff is assigned the duty of an information security officer who ensures that the use of information systems complies with the relevant data protection and privacy legislation. The person responsible for this may also have to introduce controls that ensure pre-defined access and security levels to all databases used in the organization are maintained. Databases may be classified in terms of low, medium and high sensitivity. Of course, the latter category includes patient records which are only accessible by authorized health care staff and are kept confidential under the rules of professional conduct. But also in this category are financial information, such as payroll information and payment authorization systems, as well as any other critical information, which must be protected from unauthorized alteration or disclosure. Assessment of security risks should follow a pre-defined schedule which involves periodic evaluation of the physical and administrative controls to prevent unauthorized access.

Financial controls are important for any organization. The consequences of not having financial controls become all too obvious fairly quickly: lack of accountability, funds spent inappropriately, lack of information, unexplained losses and many more. The other important thing to bear in mind is that these controls must be up to date and actually applied. All too often important documents, such as the budget manual produced to explain and specify how to prepare and monitor budgets, are rarely used and out of date. This will be no protection to the organization, or yourself and your future, when something goes wrong.

The control environment

To ensure probity an organization needs to maintain sound internal controls. These may be (high-level) organization-wide controls, or specific to certain parts or aspects of the organization (low-level controls).

If such controls are to be observed and maintained they must become part of the culture of the organization and this requires the evident commitment of the most senior management within the organization both in observing the controls and in monitoring them at the highest levels. However, controls need to be effective without stifling the scope for initiative within the organization. It should also be borne in mind that, however effective, internal controls cannot provide certainty against material errors, losses or fraud; they can only provide reasonable assurances.

High-level controls

High-level controls are designed and implemented at board level and above, for example, at district or regional level for some public sector systems. They are part of the governance system which determines the relations between the different levels of hierarchy in the organization. The means of high-level controls can be defined in various ways, for example through a corporate charter, bylaws, formal policies or rule of law.

The board of directors or governors

The duties of the board usually comprise a range of both supervisory and advisory functions and there are different models of how boards are composed.

1 Boards may include both executive and non-executive directors. Executive directors are employees of the organization with functional roles such as chief executive, finance director, director of clinical services, director of nursing. Non-executive directors are not employees of the organization. They are usually

people with relevant experience in the wider community, who are appointed as watchdogs or advisers and bring in an independent perspective which is not necessarily related to health care.

2 Other models may favour a stricter separation between top management and supervision of the organization, where executive directors are not represented at board level and the organization is supervised by a board composed of stakeholders such as financial experts from government, local politicians and representatives from professional associations, patients' associations, unions etc.

In both cases the owners, whether government or private sector, usually reserve a final say in controlling the organization. A key consideration in high-level controls is avoiding conflicts of interest which may arise from the different roles board members may occupy. Typical conflicts of interest which may interfere with the exercise of judgement could for example arise when:

*   government representatives act in both the roles of purchaser and provider;
*   non-executive directors have business relations with the organization or its competitors;
*   executive directors supervise actions they are responsible for at the operational level.

Thus it is important that a clear structure of duties and voting rights is maintained which reflects the appropriate distribution of authority and responsibility in the organization. The typical roles of a supervisory board include reviewing financial performance and advising on the strategic direction of the organization. This usually involves:

*   approval of the strategic planning, for example, the business plan which describes the objectives of the organization and financial funds needed over a period of three to five years;
*   approval and control of the budget;
*   approval of annual financial statements, balance sheet, income and cash flow statements;
*   deciding on key employees, for example the appointment of executive directors and their rules of conduct;
*   setting remuneration and evaluating performance of the chief executive and other executive directors;
*   advising or deciding on the appointment of the external auditor;
*   reviewing financial controls and overseeing internal audit.

The two latter duties are particularly relevant for the effective functioning of financial controls and they are often exercised by an independent audit committee, which liaises with the external auditor and approves internal audit reports.

External audit

Large organizations are required to appoint an independent auditor who scrutinizes the annual financial statements and produces an audit report. Those responsible for appointing the external auditor should ensure that auditors rotate at regular intervals to ensure a fresh view on the organization. It is increasingly accepted that, in order to maintain an independent position, external auditors should not perform consultancy work for the organization they audit.

A key function of the audit committee is to review the audit report and recommend appropriate actions to the board. The board will focus on any critical section of the audit report and particularly on the auditor's conclusions. In this statement the auditor expresses a judgement which according to professional standards takes the form of either a 'qualified' or 'unqualified' opinion. An unqualified opinion refers to the organization as a whole and means that the audit report reveals no major irregularities, that the financial statements represent a true and fair view of the organization and are not inconsistent with the country's generally accepted accounting principles (GAAPs) (as described in Chapter 9). If the organization is in financial troubles, a qualified opinion may be issued which disclaims (or qualifies) the report, stating the auditor's concerns about shortcomings. Concerns expressed in a disclaimer of opinion are, for example, that the report provides insufficient material evidence (scope limitations) or does not comply with GAAPs, or raises serious doubts that the organization is able to exist in the future (going concern). However, the board should not be informed about such serious financial difficulties at a relatively late stage, through the letter of the auditor, but through the early warning system of financial controls which enables the board to take corrective measures as early as possible.

Internal audit

Organizations should have an established internal audit function with responsibility for reviewing the internal controls. In overseeing internal audit it should be ensured that systems of internal control are operating effectively, that there is a strategy for preventing and detecting fraud and corruption and that the organization has a risk management strategy. The internal auditor will check whether necessary controls are in place and whether they are working satisfactorily. Much of the work of internal auditors is to test representative samples of transactions to ensure that controls are working as they should. Internal auditors may also be responsible for undertaking special investigations where fraud or corruption is suspected, and value-for-money studies. The board's audit committee should approve the planned work of the internal audit department and internal audit findings should be reported back to the committee.

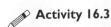 **Activity 16.3**

  1 In which ways are high-level control exercised in your organization?
  2 How might an effective system of budgetary control help to uncover mismanagement, fraud or corruption?

 Feedback

  1 There are large international variations in the design and approaches to high-level controls. In traditional hierarchies there are no boards. Controls are exercised by standing orders from the next highest level of the organization. Where boards are appointed their responsibilities may range between merely giving advice and tight financial supervision of the management. Where the advisory function prevails,

members of the board may have no financial experts and have limited insight in financial matters. In many public sector organizations, financial controls may be centralized with less responsibility given to boards of directors and in particular to non-executive directors. In these cases financial controls are within the responsibility of regional health authorities or the Ministry of Health.

2 An effective budgetary control system, particularly if budgets are devolved to operational levels, will result in the regular distribution of budget reports that are both timely and accurate and include an appropriate level of detail. Variances will be highlighted so that any deviations from planned activity will be brought to the early attention of the responsible manager who should be in a position to identify the reasons and to investigate any suspicious circumstances.

Low-level controls

Individual units or departments within the organization should all have internal financial controls designed to:

- safeguard the assets of the organization by assigning responsibility for them, ensuring that they are physically safe and insured in the event of loss;
- ensure that transactions are accurately recorded and that there is a reliable audit trail;
- authorize transactions, with authorization levels for different transactions such as purchases above a certain value being clearly established.

These internal financial controls are the responsibility of managers; they will both help to reveal genuine errors and serve to discourage fraud and corruption. To minimize the risk of fraud and corruption it is important to separate duties so that different staff members safeguard assets, record transactions and authorize transactions. Internal audit will normally be given responsibility for identifying risks, ensuring that internal control systems are in place and working, and that they are adequate. Separation of functions is particularly necessary in purchase and payment with more than one person being responsible for ordering and checking in goods, authorizing invoices for payment, issuing cheques and entering and authorizing electronic payments.

Activity 16.4 is designed to help you identify the scope for fraud and some of the checks that can help reveal it.

✎ Activity 16.4

You have been asked by your government to investigate the integrity of the low-level financial controls of a district hospital. Before starting your job you found in the records the following description of the payroll and creditor payments system. While reading, identify potential gaps in financial control which you think should be further investigated. Write a short note on each weakness you suspect, what it implies and the action that should be taken.

The *payroll* section is responsible for paying the salaries of all staff working in the hospital. Salaries are paid by direct transfer to the employee's bank account. In addition there are some temporary staff working through an agency – payment for these staff is made to the agency.

All changes to salaries, new starters and new leavers are checked by the human resources officer before being passed on to the payroll section. All changes are entered onto the computerized payroll system by the assistants or the payroll manager. As job turnover is high in support staff, leave notes are batched before amending the payroll system. Monthly salaries and changes need to be authorized on the computer system by the payroll manager before any payments are made.

Payments for agency nurses are based on timesheets. The nurse completes a weekly timesheet, gets it signed by an authorized manager and forwards it to the agency. The agency sends one invoice each month for all the nursing costs (along with copies of all timesheets) to the payroll department. The payroll department makes the payment to the agency, provided the timesheets have been authorized.

The *creditor payments* section in the finance department is responsible for processing payments for all goods and services (excluding salaries) and sending cheques out. Firms send invoices to the section for goods and services they have provided to the hospital. The invoices are matched to order forms and processed on the computerized payments system by the two payments officers. The payments manager must authorize the payments on the computer system before the cheques can be printed and sent out. In the event of both clerks being absent the payments manager can process the payments as well as authorize them. Blank cheques are stored in a safe in the financial controller's office and can only be signed out by payments section staff.

 Feedback

Compare your findings and recommendations with those in Table 16.1.

Table 16.1 Gaps in control – payroll and creditor payments systems

Weakness	Implication	Recommendation
Agency nursing staff are responsible for handing in their timesheets once they have been approved by the manager who does not keep a copy	Agency staff could amend the hours worked after the timesheet has been approved	Managers employing agency staff should keep copies of all timesheets. Periodic checks should be made to ensure that submitted timesheets agree with the copies retained
The payroll manager can both enter and authorize payroll details for new employees	Inadequate separation of duties – there is no independent check of payroll details entered by the payroll manager	When the payroll manager enters payroll details onto the system these should be authorized by another senior member of staff
Batching of leave notes causes delays in removing employees from the payroll	Delays in removing leavers may result in incorrect payment of salary and the costs of recovering overpayments	All leavers should be promptly removed from the payroll once notification has been received

Invoices are not matched with goods received notes before payment is authorized	Lack of evidence that the goods have been received	Matching of order forms with good received notes or any other evidence that the good or service has been delivered before processing for payment

Summary

There is wide scope for maladministration, fraud and corruption in health care as in many other sectors. The increasing use of IT has resulted in the need for measures that will prevent a range of fraudulent behaviours including fraud, theft of data and of software, hacking and the introduction of viruses. Sound internal controls are necessary both at:

- high level, where executive and non-executive directors should be actively involved in promoting and observing controls; they should ensure that the organization complies with regulations imposed by external funding bodies, that an effective budgetary control system is in place and that there is an adequate internal audit function;
- low level, where sound operational controls must be in place and observed in order to minimize the risk of fraud.

References

Calderon, T.G. and Green, B.P. (1994) Internal fraud leaves its mark, *National Public Accountant*, August: 17–19 and 36–8.

OECD (Organization for Economic Cooperation and Development) (2003) *Development Assistance Committee Network on Governance: Synthesis of Lessons Learned of Donor Practices in Fighting Corruption*. Paris: OECD.

Transparency International (2004) *Global Corruption Report*. London: Pluto Press.

Weiner, M. (1962) *The Policy of Scarcity: Public Press and Political Response in India*. Chicago: University of Chicago.

17 Accountability and regulatory control

Overview

This chapter reviews how governance and regulation is used to set objectives for financial management and ensure that the organization achieves those objectives. Whether these objectives are specified in government regulations or set by the organization itself, as discussed in the previous chapter, the need for governance and regulation and the principles for achieving it are the same. For you this has significance too, because you work in an environment that is regulated to some degree either by the government or self-regulated by the organization; the extent to which this is successful or not impacts directly on you. In this chapter you will examine how health care organizations are regulated and draw out the general principles of the need for financial regulation and the benefits of regulation. When you have completed this chapter you will have an overview of regulatory principles and how these apply for your organization.

Learning objectives

By the end of this chapter you should be able to:

- outline approaches to regulation in the health sector
- give examples of regulations applying to financial management
- explain the principles of corporate governance
- explain basic approaches to financial control (through structure, policies and procedures) and identify how these are applied in your organization

Key terms

Corporate governance Structures and functions describing the distribution of rights and responsibilities within an organization and the rules for decision-making among the different participants, such as the board, managers, owners or government.

Financial directions Rules and procedures describing the key financial responsibilities of the financial director and of the chief executive officer.

Hierarchy of control The combination of regulations and procedures to ensure openness, integrity and accountability in running an organization.

Job description A document defining the level of authority, responsibility and accountability of a job.

Regulation Government intervention to achieve specific objectives in the health sector through legal controls and incentives.

Standing orders Rules that are permanently in force, outlining the general terms of managing the organization.

Governance and regulation

Consider the following two scenarios about two extremes of government behaviour towards hospitals, as described by Busse et al (2002):

1 In the first scenario any entrepreneur has a right to set up a hospital, determine how to run it and be responsible for all losses and profit. The private owner would set price levels, decide on all salaries and have absolute freedom in business relations with suppliers and other health care organizations including mergers and takeovers.
2 In the second scenario only government can establish hospitals, patients are not charged for services and the annually allocated funds cover all costs. Salaries are paid according to public sector tariffs and the hospital has no independent financial position in relation to suppliers or to other hospitals.

Both scenarios describe an unregulated situation: the first, because no restrictions are imposed to control the economic behaviour of the provider; the second, because government itself acts as owner of the hospital and sets its own rules through governance. While a *laissez-faire* approach as described in the first scenario is rarely used even in countries with extensive private health care markets, the second scenario is not uncommon where the public sector is also the main provider of health care and is directly responsible for managing hospitals. But in many settings the actual governance structure lies between the two extremes.

Regulation can be defined as a government intervention which involves legislation to achieve specific objectives in the health sector that would otherwise not be achieved. Regulatory mechanisms include two basic principles:

• legal controls, which are enforced by sanctions if the objectives are not met;
• incentives, which aim to influence the behaviour of providers in such a way that desired outcomes are achieved.

Regulation is used to set minimum standards for organizations not only of a financial nature but also to achieve social goals in the functioning of hospitals. Often legislation enacts a set of basic requirements that extends to both public and private providers whereas more specific ones may apply to those receiving public funding.

✐ Activity 17.1

Assume you have been asked to assist in designing regulations for hospitals. Which areas should be covered and which minimum standards should be set in general and with particular respect to financial issues?

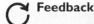 **Feedback**

> You may have found a range of social and financial objectives that can be implemented through regulation. Regulatory control may cover location, size, range of services offered and the obligation to treat all patients. Minimum standards may be set for the qualification of staff, skills mix and quality of services provided. Financial objectives include pricing, the use of any surplus, procedures for market entry (capital and security requirements) and exit (rules for mergers and acquisitions to prevent monopolies).

Regulation and dissemination of accounting standards

The starting point of regulation is often a strong interest in self-regulation of professional groups. This also applies to financial bodies agreeing on accounting principles and standards. Rules which have initially been agreed by professional bodies may later be enacted into legislation or adopted by regulating authorities. Generally, two philosophies of regulating the requirements for accounting can be distinguished:

1   The British and US approach which is widely used in the English-speaking world and is based on the Anglo-Saxon law tradition. Only basic requirements are regulated by law. Standards are further developed by jurisdiction and by professional bodies. The key focus is protecting investments rather than creditors. Tax assessment is not included in the financial statements.
2   The Continental European approach, which is based on the Roman law tradition and which focuses mainly on protecting creditors and safeguarding the capital employed. All requirements of the financial statements are codified in detail and regulated by law, and professional bodies do not play a major role in standard-setting. The balance sheet also includes the assessment of taxes.

Thus accounting standards differ widely and international organizations in health care may have to produce different sets of financial reports, depending on where they operate.

A number of international organizations such as the EU and the World Bank have addressed this problem and supported the harmonization of national accounting standards. Since 1973 the International Accounting Standards Committee (IASC) has also played an important role in promulgating standards and interpretations for accounting. As you read in Chapter 1, an increasing number of countries require organizations to comply with these.

However, for public services in many countries, implementing accounting standards is still a challenge. In recent years many low- and middle-income countries have moved from simple cash accounting to the more complex accrual accounting which takes into consideration the value of assets and liabilities. While accrual accounting gives a better picture of the financial status of an organization there are number of restrictions to implementation (Athukorala and Reid 2003):

1   In many low-income countries there is a shortage of qualified accountants in the public sector and limits in IT infrastructure inhibit the dissemination of more sophisticated methods.

2 Where government has to deal with different donor agencies, conflicting objectives and methodologies may reduce the coherence of the approach. Donor consortia and international agencies have addressed this issue and increasingly support the use of common standards and reporting requirements.

3 There is a lack of corporate governance and of a business culture to support the introduction of quality accounting and auditing standards. It has also been argued that attempts to improve government transparency and accountability may threaten the income of politicians and bureaucrats.

Overall it appears to be better to have a simple but functioning accounting system rather than a more complex one that is not accepted or requires an inappropriately high input of management capacity to run effectively. To be accepted at the level of policy-makers and senior officials, improvements should be actively promoted and the advantage of proper financial reporting for decision-making in public services should be made clear.

 Activity 17.2

Find out how the requirements for financial reporting are regulated in public sector organizations in your country.

 Feedback

You may have identified the professional body responsible or the law governing accounting standards in public sector organizations in your country. Depending on the environment and historical traditions, different standards and frameworks may be used. Internationally, a strong trend of convergence of accounting systems can be observed, which may have caused recent reforms in your country.

Corporate governance

Corporate governance is the system by which business corporations are directed and controlled. The corporate governance structure specifies the distribution of rights and responsibilities among different participants in the corporation, such as the board, managers, shareholders and other stakeholders, and spells out the rules and procedures for making decisions on corporate affairs. By doing this, it also provides the structure through which the company objectives are set, and the means of attaining those objectives and monitoring performance.

(Cadbury Report 1992)

Issues of corporate governance attract public attention if something goes wrong. In the UK in the 1980s high-profile financial scandals and the questionable conduct of public officials in certain circumstances led to an increasing lack of confidence in public and private sector organizations. As a result, a commission was set up to investigate the issue of corporate governance and to make recommendations to ensure that company directors act in the interest of their shareholders. The report was highly influential in developing the structure and process of good governance and provided a general definition which has been widely accepted and also applied to public sector organizations.

The principles on which its recommendations were based have general relevance not only to organizations in the UK but to all organizations in which the owners do not directly exercise control. The principles have been further developed in the international context by an initiative led by the Organization for Economic Cooperation and Development (OECD) and were also influential in shaping the governance of public sector organizations under a policy of new public sector management in many countries. Corporate governance operates on several key principles (Bhatta 2003; OECD 2004):

1 A clear distinction exists between ownership and management. In health care organizations this may be reflected in the separation of supervisory and operational functions. Where applicable a separation is also maintained between providing and financing health care.
2 Clear objectives are in place which cover not only financial targets but also health care goals such as those related to equity of access and the volume and quality of the services provided.
3 Performance standards are set and linked with appropriate incentives encouraging management to achieve planned goals.
4 Accountability is the key concept by which management is held responsible for its actions. It is the ability to stand up to scrutiny, public judgement and professional codes of conduct. Management is answerable to the board and individual members of staff are regarded as accountable for their decisions and actions in their areas of responsibility.
5 Thus, following from the above, openness and integrity are central values of good governance. Openness relates to promoting confidence in the organization, disclosure and transparency of information. Integrity requires straightforward dealing as well as completeness and ethical use of information. Other principles of ethical conduct include selflessness, honesty, probity and objectivity.

A statement acknowledging the principles of corporate governance and the directors' responsibilities as well as what they are doing to meet these responsibilities is increasingly included in the annual report and accounts of both private and public sector organizations.

Implementing governance structures and procedures

In implementing governance structures most countries have enacted laws which not only set rules for public hospitals but also for any health care organization that receives public money, such as NGOs or private providers which have contracts with public financing agencies. A distinction can be made between internal and external accountability of management:

• external accountability is the monitoring of performance against plans, and includes activity levels, value for money, quality and financial management reports;
• internal accountability includes the hierarchy of budgets, clinical audit and the full range of self-regulated local policies and procedures that are in place.

All activities relevant to accountability have to be clearly documented to provide transparency and openness of the governance structure and procedures. Such documents should outline how a hospital operates and the controls performed (Mellet *et al.* 1993), including:

- *Standing orders:* formulated by the board and outlining the general terms of managing the hospital and the principles governing the actions of each employee.
- *Financial directions:* describing the key financial responsibilities of the financial director and of the chief executive officer.
- *Standing financial instructions:* containing more detailed information on the conduct expected from management in financial issues.
- *The financial control system:* clearly defining the flow of responsibility at each stage of the process and the safeguards for integrity of the financial information. Tools that help implement financial control at each level of the organization should be written procedures and checklists.

Job descriptions tie in here as a further means of documentation, since they provide a detailed description of the tasks assigned to each employee. The job descriptions correspond with the financial control hierarchy and specifically reflect the different levels of:

- *authority:* the right to give directions to other staff;
- *responsibility:* the obligation to carry out defined actions;
- *accountability:* the obligation to report back to the next higher level.

This ensures that no doubt is left about the limits of power and influence of each element of the financial control hierarchy.

Governance of public sector organizations does not only cover accountability and financial controls but also a wide range of other issues related to planning, human resource management, external financing and the dealings with any surplus or deficit. The overall aim is to ensure that managers operate in line with government policy and meet required targets. Thus, managers are required to follow certain rules and procedures. For example, the details of the planning cycle as well as various constraints to planning will be prescribed by the government. Planning rules will also cover mid-term planning to demonstrate financial viability over a planning period of three to five years. The strategic business plan of the organization must tie in with both its operational plans and the wider planning at central level. To be able to reconcile the planning information from different organizations with the strategic plan, for example, the government five-year plan for the health sector, a range of conditions should be met to ensure that:

- source and volume of financing follow agreed patterns of resource allocation;
- services provided and activity levels are in line with government priorities;
- income and expenditure of the organization tie in with government revenue and spending plans;
- capital expenditure over several years is reconciled with government capital planning;
- assumptions on inflation, interest rates and economic growth are applied in a uniform way.

Once the mid-term plans are approved by the central authority, the organization will derive from this the detailed plan for the current and coming year and be held responsible for implementing it and monitoring activity to ensure that it is achieved (Mellet *et al.* 1993).

Activity 17.3

1   Briefly summarize the governance structure of your organization. This is probably best done by means of a diagram or chart.
2   Indicate the hierarchy of control that applies in your organization.
3   Describe the procedures for mid-term financial planning in your organization.

Feedback

1 The governance structure normally includes a carefully defined range of responsibilities which can be displayed in an organization chart. It will describe to whom the acting persons/bodies are responsible, what powers they have in decision-making and what is expected of their performance and how this is assessed.

2 The hierarchy of control will range from broad policy statements of what is required to detailed procedures that must be followed to deliver the performance standards specified by the policy. For instance, a policy statement requiring 'the safeguarding of assets' will include detailed procedures on what to do to record assets and procedures on how equipment should be transferred between one department and another.

3 Business plans aim to demonstrate financial viability of an organization in the future and they cover a foreseeable period of time of three to five years. In decentralized organizations individual plans need to align with the overall strategy of the organization. Reconciliation is achieved by planning rules and common assumptions of key factors set by the centre.

Summary

Government may enact regulation to ensure that, among other goals, minimum standards in financial reporting and control are maintained. Increasingly, international accounting standards are adopted and a range of international actors are involved in improving the quality of financial reports and promoting best practice in accounting. Corporate governance is concerned with ensuring that those who run public and private organizations display openness, integrity and accountability. These principles are increasingly used in public sector organizations and implemented and controlled by a combination of regulations and procedures, which form part of the hierarchy of control. The governance structure is designed to agree the general terms by which the business of the organization is conducted and to ensure that agreed strategic objectives are achieved.

References

Athukorala, S.L. and Reid, B. (2003) *Accrual Budgeting and Accounting in Government and its Relevance for Developing Member Countries*. Manila: ADB.

Bhatta, G. (2003) *Post-NPM Themes in Public Sector Governance State Services*. Commission Working Paper No. 17. Wellington, NZ: State Services Commission.

Busse, R., van der Grinten, T. and Svensson, P-G. (2002) Regulating entrepreneurial behaviour in hospitals: theory and practice in *Regulating entrepreneurial behaviour in European health care systems*.

Cadbury Report (1992) *Report of the Committee on the Financial Aspects of Corporate Governance*. London: Gee & Co. Ltd.

Mellett, H., Marriott, N. and Harries, S. (1993) *Financial Management in the NHS: A Manager's Handbook*. London: Chapman & Hall.

OECD (Organization for Economic Cooperation and Development) (2004) *Principles of Corporate Governance*. Paris: OECD.

18	# Managing performance

Overview

This chapter reviews information needs for managing performance. In Chapter 14 you looked at financial performance ratios and their use and limitations in interpreting financial statements. Now you will look at how this information can be integrated with other approaches to performance management. The chapter discusses the information needs for continuously monitoring performance and the purpose, use and limitations of financial and non-financial performance measures. A frequently used approach is the efficiency index which you will explore in further detail in the chapter. Finally the chapter presents the balanced scorecard approach as a comprehensive and frequently used framework for evaluating and managing performance.

Learning objectives

By the end of this chapter you should be able to:

- **use appropriate non-financial and financial measures of performance**
- **discuss the efficiency index and how to interpret it**
- **identify more wide-ranging applications for the efficiency index in your organization**
- **describe the balanced scorecard approach in relation to health care organizations**

Key terms

Balanced scorecard A systematic approach to performance management, focusing not only on financial targets but also on customer needs, internal processes, learning and innovation.

Efficiency index A performance indicator combining the change of activity with the corresponding change of costs.

Lagging measures Historical indicators that inform on past performance.

Leading measures Future-directed indicators that a specific outcome is likely to be achieved.

Performance indicators Financial and non-financial measures used for monitoring activity levels, efficiency and quality of service provision by comparing actual with expected results.

Changing information needs

All organizations operate in a dynamic environment where they must adapt in order to survive. In many health systems, whether or not there is a profit motive, there is a concerted movement towards more market-oriented approaches in the belief that they will enable organizations to identify potential cost savings and so allocate limited resources more efficiently. In large and complex organizations these trends call for the effective use of sophisticated management information systems in preparing detailed costing of services and monitoring performance against these costings, and new approaches to improving efficiency.

This approach implies that performance can be measured and reasonably controlled by management and that those responsible are accountable for their actions. Performance measures need to be reliable and valid and can comprise a range of both qualitative and quantitative data. However, the figures do not tell much about the causes underlying changes in performance. Performance measures need an analytical context to be understood; for example, a change in vaccination rate among children under 5 could be due to a range of demand and supply factors.

A key approach to measuring performance is to analyse changes in performance over time or to compare performance with other providers or absolute standards. Suppose as a board member you are confronted with a range of financial and non-financial performance indicators. In interpreting any current financial information you would compare it to the budget and to last year's accounts. You may also look up the relevant strategic plan such as a business plan over three years to assess the long-term expectations of the organization. You may also use other organizations' aggregated district or regional data with which to compare your organization's performance. Before making any conclusions you would ensure that the information is presented consistently for the same items and the same period of time, and you would also need to know what tolerance (deviation from the plan) is acceptable. The latter requires some knowledge of the context.

Non-financial performance indicators

Most people interested in the performance of health services are not primarily interested in financial performance. They are more likely to want to know how the service has performed in terms of the outcomes of treatment, how long patients have to wait for treatment, numbers of operations performed, occupancy of beds etc. With IT support, health care organizations are now able to routinely produce a range of non-financial performance indicators. While most of these are used for management purposes, some may be required as part of the regulatory framework within which the organization operates. Data on costs associated with defined workload activity can be recorded to compare performance across a region or the country as a whole.

These measures may include, for example:

- measures of activity such as the number of inpatient discharges, day cases and accident and emergency attendances;
- value-for-money measures – the bed occupancy rate, average length of stay and theatre utilization;

- quality measures – waiting times for outpatient appointments and the number of cancelled outpatient sessions.

 Activity 18.1

1 List the non-financial performance indicators that are relevant to your organization.
2 What are the potential problems of using performance indicators for comparisons across organizations?

 Feedback

1 You may have identified indicators such as:

- complaints
- waiting time for first appointments
- waiting lists
- post-operative mortality

2 While performance indicators are useful within the organization, their use for comparisons requires that standards of measurement are clearly defined and maintained. It must be ensured that the data are timely and accurate and are based on the same definitions to be able to compare like with like. They should not be used in situations where a different case-mix may make comparison meaningless. Often differences are poorly understood and can only be interpreted with additional contextual information. Another key problem is that many of the performance indicators do not focus on outcomes. They say much about resources used and activity levels but little about the effect of this activity on health.

 Activity 18.2

Now consider financial performance. Suppose you are asked to compare the performance of a group of private sector hospitals with a group of public hospitals. You have read a report describing financial performance targets of the private sector group under each of the following headings:

a) Pricing policy
b) Break-even performance
c) Financial return
d) External financing

From what you have learned in previous chapters, explain why these concepts are important and how they would translate into assessing financial performance of the public sector hospitals.

 Feedback

You may have found that there are some limits in applying these performance targets to public sector hospitals, particularly where these are directly managed units within the government hierarchy. Nevertheless with some adaptations to the specific conditions in public sector hospitals they can be applied in a meaningful way, as the following examples show:

a) Clearly, for a private organization, pricing strategies are key to making profits. However, pricing decisions also matter in the public sector, particularly under internal market arrangements. For example, it is important that provisions for medical negligence and other such items are recognized in the cost structure. The hospital would average provisions over a number of years rather than attempting to recover these as the provisions are incurred. Averaging will tend to stabilize prices. If averaging were not applied then prices would be erratic and could fluctuate wildly from year to year.

b) Break-even analysis is an absolute requirement not only in the private sector to assess the starting point for profits but also in public sector hospitals to ensure costs are recovered and that spending is not excessive.

c) Financial returns can be measured in various ways. In the private sector financial ratios such as the ROCE (discussed in Chapter 14) are frequently used to summarize overall financial performance. In public sector organizations measures considering returns on assets are less common but can be used as a requirement to demonstrate that the net assets are used effectively by the hospital.

d) External financing targets are needed to manage the debt burden of an organization. Unlike private hospitals which can assess the capital market, public sector organizations usually operate under strict external financing limits. This can, in effect, be a limit on the strategic development of the organization. In many countries public sector organizations may be allowed under defined conditions to borrow money. However, usually new funding is only available as part of an agreed long-term strategic plan, which would be closely monitored.

Efficiency index

The *efficiency index* is a useful and versatile indicator of performance. The index works by relating the change in the level of activity to the impact of this change on costs. The way in which the index is calculated is shown in Figure 18.1.

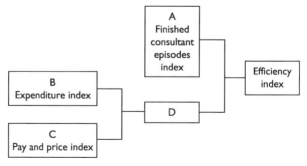

Figure 18.1 Calculation of the efficiency index

Source: Mellet *et al.* (1993)

The index compares the rate of increase of activity measured in finished consultant episodes (FCEs) with the rate of increase of expenses and the pay and price index. The first step is the calculation of the rate of increase of expenses and the pay and price index. Whether the rate of increase of expenses is higher or lower than the rate of increase of the pay and price index does not indicate whether performance is improving or declining. The relative change in expenses compared with the pay and price index needs to be compared with output to decide this. Figure 18.2 shows how to interpret the efficiency index.

	Output index lower than combined expenditure and pay and price index	Output index higher than combined expenditure and pay and price index
Expenditure index higher than pay and price index	Efficiency declining	Efficiency improving
Expenditure index lower than pay and price index	Efficiency declining	Efficiency improving

Figure 18.2 Interpreting the efficiency index

Activity 18.3

Calculate the efficiency index for a district hospital using Table 18.1. Assume an inflation index of 2.8 per cent for the year.

Table 18.1 Efficiency index (data)

	2005	2006
Activity		
Accident and emergency	80 000	78 000
Inpatients	50 000	53 000
Day cases	20 000	20 600
Total	150 000	151 600
Expenses		
Operating expenses ($000)	150 000	163 000

Feedback

The calculations for the efficiency index are shown in Table 18.2.

The efficiency index shows that overall costs are increasing at a rate of 4 per cent faster than activity (100 per cent – 96 per cent). Alternatively, activities are increasing at a rate that is 4 per cent slower than costs. Possible reasons for this should be further investigated. An analysis may reveal waste or inefficient use of resources or improvements in service quality without matching activity gains.

Table 18.2 Efficiency index (calculations)

	2005	2006	Index
Activity			
Accident and emergency	80 000	78 000	
Inpatients	50 000	53 000	
Day cases	20 000	20 600	
Total	150 000	151 600	
Activity index (A)			1.011
Expenses			
Operating expenses ($000)	150 000	163 000	
Operating expenses index (B)			1.087
Inflation index (C)			1.028
Expenses index/inflation index (D)			1.057
Efficiency index (A/D)			0.96

The efficiency index is a useful concept because it is a way of assessing performance that directly relates activities to costs. This is helpful as a way of viewing costs because:

- increased revenue does not always follow increased activity; the efficiency index highlights this and can be used to justify the need for extra funding;
- in many cases revenue data may not be available, for instance for internal support departments, but activity and cost data are available; the efficiency index can be used to justify current spending and justify the need for extra funding without revenue statistics.

The efficiency index can be applied in almost any part of the organization whether it has income or not, just so long as activity data are available.

Activity 18.4

As a manager it is a good exercise in flexible thinking to identify as many areas as you can where this type of index could be applied in your organization. List these in Table 18.3 with examples of the activity data that can be incorporated in an efficiency index.

Table 18.3 Possible applications for the efficiency index

Department where the efficiency index could be applied	Units of measurement for activities to be included in the index

Feedback

There should be many examples where the efficiency index can be applied, including support departments. The length of your list should indicate the potential and value of this versatile performance measure. It is certainly worth considering whether you can use this in your unit for the future.

The balanced scorecard

A key problem with the methods you have considered so far is that they only measure past performance and are not integrated with the strategic management of the organization. The *balanced scorecard (BSC)* is an approach which addresses these shortcomings and puts a strong emphasis on translating the long-term strategic goals of the organization into operational objectives which then can be implemented and controlled in a systematic way (Kaplan and Norton 1996).

The approach was originally developed for private business and has since spread to the public sector and not-for-profit organizations, with the primary focus shifting from financial goals, such as profitability, to non-financial goals related to the organization's mission. For example, in applying the BSC to health care organizations, the concept has been modified to reflect the specific realities of the sector and to integrate efficiency with quality of service provision (Zelman *et al.* 2003).

The methodology evolves in several steps from a general strategic view of the organization to more operational detail. The basic idea is that all of the organization's systems should be in line with achieving the organization's mission. This requires that a common vision of the purpose and primary aims of the organization is shared and actively communicated among staff.

First, the key strategies necessary to realize the vision are identified. This step is not just a list of strategies but requires a systematic analysis which identifies the critical strategic objectives in relation to four different views or perspectives (Kaplan and Norton 1996):

- *The financial perspective:* which financial goals must be achieved in order to be able to fulfil our mission?
- *The customer perspective:* which needs of our customers (patients, stakeholders) must be met to be able to achieve our organizational goals?
- *The process perspective:* how should we develop our internal processes and in what areas should we excel in meeting our customers' needs and our financial goals?
- *Learning and innovation:* what capacities do we need to enhance internal processes? How should the organization change in terms of infrastructure and technology and what skills and competencies do we need to improve our services?

Figure 18.3 illustrates the four perspectives of the balanced scorecard in relation to the organization, its mission and its vision and strategy. The different perspectives

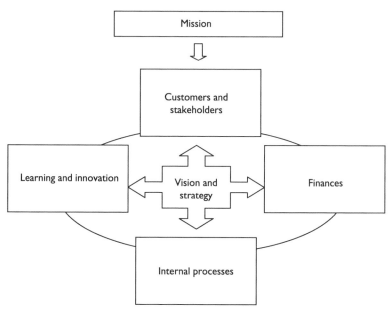

Figure 18.3 The balanced scorecard

can be more easily understood if you relate them to the people acting in and around the organization (Rohm 2004). The financial perspective relates to the owners of the organization as represented, for example, by government, NGOs or shareholders of private companies. The customer perspective represents not only the view of patients but also of any other internal or external customer or stakeholder. The process perspective is seen through the eyes of those held accountable for the functioning of the organization. So these are managers as well as any other process owner, for example, clinicians in their individual area of responsibility. The learning and innovation perspective is represented by the employees' creativity and readiness to develop new skills and competencies to be able to meet organizational needs.

A key point which makes a well designed BSC different from a random collection of performance indicators is that the measures should be balanced appropriately to reflect the right mix of:

- *subjective and objective measures:* for example, survey data on customer and employee satisfaction and objective data such as occupancy, cases treated, financial ratios etc.;
- *lagging and leading measures:* lagging measures are historical indicators that inform on past performance; leading measures are future-directed indicating that a specific outcome is likely to be achieved.

It is also important that the four perspectives are linked with each other and form a logical sequence: innovation and process are the drivers for change – the customer and financial perspectives are the outcomes resulting from these drivers. For example, mobilizing funds through a rural health insurance scheme (the financial perspective) requires that patients and stakeholders in the community are satisfied with the quality of the services provided and therefore willing to pay the contribution (customer perspective). To provide the quality of service demanded and to be able to collect revenue, management must improve its clinical and administrative processes (process perspective). This in turn requires appropriate training of staff and the implementation of financial control systems (learning and innovation). Thus the links between the four perspectives should be understood as a chain of cause and effect relationships.

In breaking down the strategic goals to the operative level, the practical design of the BSC takes the following four steps (Kaplan and Norton 1996):

1 *Deciding on key objectives:* for each of the perspectives three to four main strategic objectives, which are critical for success, are identified and agreed upon. This step and the following ones should be carried out in a team involving participation of staff from the relevant areas.
2 *Designing the measurement architecture:* for each of the objectives the appropriate measure is agreed. Routine measures may not be adequate and often organizations develop their own specific measures.
3 *Setting targets:* the target to be achieved is agreed for each of the objectives, together with the appropriate planning period.
4 *Deciding on the implementation plan:* finally, for each objective the appropriate initiative or action is agreed, and decisions are reached as to how the results will be integrated in the organization's management information system and the planning cycle.

The approach of the BSC can be used at both the central level of the organization and in departments and sub-units. However, it is important that targets agreed at lower levels fit in with the central strategy (see Figure 18.4). By this process of cascading, that is, devolving central strategic objectives into appropriate numbers of specific targets, the congruence of goals is maintained between the different levels of the organization.

The BSC is a performance management and measurement system with a range of advantages compared to simple collections of performance measures. It has a

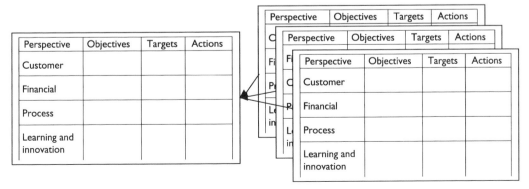

Figure 18.4 Cascading the balanced score card

strong focus on communication and behavioural change. It enables managers to combine strategic with operational control and to link quantitative with qualitative data. The approach is highly versatile and can be adapted to a range of settings and issues. Depending on the organizational context you can add or omit perspectives as appropriate or chose either the financial or the customer perspective as the main focus of interest. The BSC is a means of communicating a common vision and strategy so that all employees are aware of the critical issues on which to focus.

On the other hand, lack of strategy makes the BSC meaningless. The concept of goal alignment requires that a shared vision is built and this can be a challenge in organizations that are dominated by the interests of professional groups. It should also be realized that the approach is time-consuming and costly and may involve external consultants to set up the system. Also, misinterpretations and distortions may occur if the scorecard is unbalanced in that, for example, too many lagging measures are used as compared to leading ones or there is an overemphasis on objective over subjective measures. The targets should not oversimplify the complexity of management decisions. Neither should they be set too low, nor be so unrealistic as to cause opportunistic behaviour by those whose performance is assessed.

Activity 18.4

For your own organization or unit identify three important strategic objectives. For each, analyse the cause-effect relationships between the four BSC perspectives. Use the format shown in Table 18.4 and outline the appropriate performance measures, targets and actions.

Table 18.4 BSC example: improving hospital hygiene

Perspective	Objectives	Measures	Targets			Actions
			Y1	Y2	Y3	
Customers	Organizational growth through satisfied customers	Proportion of patients satisfied with treatment and cleanliness of hospital	80%	83%	86%	Survey
Financial	Increase surplus by reducing costs of hospital infections. Use surplus to increase customer satisfaction	Save on drug budget	6%	10%	13%	Monitor infection-related costs and decide on use of surplus
		Proportion of surplus reinvested in quality improvements	20%	25%	28%	
Internal processes	Strengthen infection control practices	Percentage of drug resistant hospital acquired infections	10%	5%	2%	Set up surveillance team

Learning and innovation	Raise awareness of hospital hygiene procedures	Percentage of staff trained	50%	70%	95%	Initiate cleaner hospital project. Design and implement training programme

 Feedback

Your BSC will look different depending on the objectives you have identified for your organization. It is important that you keep the design simple and understandable. Normally you will sit down as a team and think how to achieve your goals through the objectives and targets you have chosen. You will have found that the relationship between the perspectives is reciprocal. While serving customer needs will help achieving financial stability, financial success is a prerequisite of accomplishing consumer satisfaction. While target-setting is widely used in health services management, for example, in health promotion, the BSC approach has some specific features that make it a versatile performance measurement framework for financial management.

Summary

Increasingly managers in health care organizations have to make decisions that require both financial awareness and management information systems that deliver the right information in the right format at the right time. Health care organizations are often required to publish a range of financial and non-financial performance indicators. The efficiency index provides a means of comparing changes in activity levels with changes in costs. The balanced scorecard approach enables managers to translate objectives into performance targets that are reviewed from four perspectives: customers, finance, the internal processes and learning and innovation.

References

Kaplan, R. and Norton, D. (1996) Using the balanced scorecard as a strategic management system, *Harvard Business Review*, January–February: 75–85.

Mellet, H., Marriott, N. and Harries, S. (1993) *Financial Management in the NHS: A Manager's Handbook*. London: Chapman & Hall

Rohm, H. (2004) A balancing act, *Perform*, 2(2).

Zelman, W.N., Pink, G.H. and Matthias, C.B. (2003) Use of the balanced scorecard in health care, *Journal of Health Care Finance*, 29(4): 1–16.

Capital investment appraisal

Overview

In this chapter you will learn some basic techniques for capital investment appraisal so that, even if you are not able to undertake the detailed calculations, you understand the principles on which they are based and are able to select the most appropriate technique for appraising the investment you are considering.

Learning objectives

By the end of this chapter you should be able to:

- discuss the need for capital investment appraisal
- describe the uses and limitations of the payback method and the average rate of return
- use discounted cash flow techniques to calculate the net present value and the internal rate of return of capital investments

Key terms

Average rate of return A measure of profitability allowing investments with different capital outlays to be compared. The average rate of return is calculated as the ratio of the average cash inflow to the amount invested.

Discounted cash flow A method of comparing the profitability of alternative investments which takes the time value of money into account.

Discounting A method for adjusting the value of costs and outcomes which occur in different time periods into a common time period, usually the present.

Discount rate The rate at which future costs and outcomes are discounted to account for time preference.

Internal rate of return The discount rate where the net present value is zero.

Net present value The present value minus the initial capital outlay. If it is negative it is not worth pursuing the project.

Payback method An appraisal technique evaluating how long it will take to repay the initial investment.

Present value The amount of money that a stream of cash inflows receivable in the future is currently worth. Future cash flows are multiplied by a defined discount factor to obtain the present value.

The need for information

As a manager in a health service there will be times when you are involved in deciding whether to replace an old motor vehicle, when to update computer hardware, whether to acquire a new and expensive item of equipment, or even to build a new wing of a hospital. Decisions such as these are not everyday operating decisions. They may have big cost implications and deciding on one course of action may prevent you from expanding in some other direction. They should be guided by the principles of prudence, affordability and sustainability and be part of the long-term overall planning of the capital and revenue budget (CIPFA 2002). To make such decisions you will want to have all the necessary facts to hand. The information you will need includes:

- estimated costs of a particular course of action;
- anticipated returns from that course of action;
- other (qualitative) factors that need to be taken into account.

An approach that is frequently used for larger projects, such as new health programmes or the introduction of a new technology, is *economic evaluation*. It gives guidance on the benefits of new technologies and requires a careful assessment of all costs and consequences from a societal viewpoint. For capital investment decisions in the organizational context, *investment appraisal* techniques are more appropriate.

What is investment appraisal?

Investment appraisal techniques are based on the assumption that the main aim of a capital investment project is to generate a return on the investment. In the private sector, profitability is the most important measure of the financial acceptability of decisions. In the public sector, where profit is not the dominant motive, returns are assessed to examine whether the investment is worthwhile and increases value for money. Thus in the public sector financial decisions are judged on their ability to increase efficiency.

There are three elements that determine the return on an investment:

- the sum invested;
- returns on the sum invested;
- the lifetime of the project.

Each of the methods you will be studying takes these into account. These methods range from the very simple payback method to more sophisticated methods that take into account the time profile of the returns.

The payback method

This method establishes how long it will take to repay the initial investment. It assumes that the shorter the payback period the better the project. For example, three projects each costing $10,000 are being considered but it is decided to choose the project with the shortest payback period.

Table 19.1 Calculating the payback period

	Project A ($)	Project B ($)	Project C ($)
Initial cost	(10 000)	(10 000)	(10 000)
Year 1 projected cash receipts	5 000	2 000	3 000
Year 2 projected cash receipts	5 000	4 000	3 000
Year 3 projected cash receipts	1 000	4 000	3 000
Year 4 projected cash receipts	nil	4 000	3 000

From Table 19.1 you can see that the $10,000 initial capital outlay will be recovered within two years for Project A, three years for Project B and only during the fourth year for Project C. Project A has the shortest payback period and will therefore be chosen.

This method is used where the early return of funds is of prime importance – for example, where an organization has liquidity problems or has the capital funds earmarked for another project within two or three years' time.

You may have noticed in the example that, although Project A had the shortest payback period, if you looked at returns over the four-year period, Project B would appear to give the better return. Why, though, should you look only at four years and not an even longer period?

 Activity 19.1

Consider the following alternative capital investments both requiring an initial capital outlay of $100,000.

- Project 1 has expected returns of $20,000, $20,000, $20,000 and $50,000 in years 1 to 4 respectively
- Project 2 has expected returns of $50,000, $20,000, $20,000 and $20,000 in years 1 to 4 respectively

Use the payback method to help you recommend an investment and then comment briefly on any problems that you see with using this method.

 Feedback

The payback period for both projects is the same (four years). However, you may have noted that Project 2 yields far greater returns in the early years and would therefore be a more attractive investment. The payback method does not take any account of the time value of cash flows.

Average rate of return

Here the concern is simply with expressing profitability as an average rate of return (ARR) on the capital investment. It is calculated as follows:

$$\text{Average rate of return} = \frac{\text{average annual returns}}{\text{initial investment}} \times 100$$

For example, an organization is considering which of three projects to invest in. Cost, expected returns and lengths of the projects are summarized in Table 19.2. In this case project F is seen to yield the better rate of return. This method enables you to make a more meaningful comparison of investments with different capital outlays. A significant limitation is that it averages the profits over the time being considered so that, like the payback method, it does not take the time value of returns into account.

Table 19.2 Calculating the average rate of return

	Project D ($)	Project E ($)	Project F ($)
Initial cost	(10 000)	(18 000)	(20 000)
Year 1 projected cash receipts	3 000	9 000	8 000
Year 2 projected cash receipts	6 000	9 000	10 000
Year 3 projected cash receipts	6 000	6 000	12 000
Year 4 projected cash receipts	3 000	4 000	10 000
Total projected cash receipts	18 000	28 000	40 000
Profit over four years	8 000	10 000	20 000
Average annual profit	2 000	2 500	5 000
Average rate of return	20%	13.9%	25%

✎ Activity 19.2

Calculate the ARR for Projects A, B and C in Table 19.1, the payback method example. These figures are repeated for you in Table 19.3.

Table 19.3 The ARR for Projects A, B and C

	Project A ($)	Project B ($)	Project C ($)
Initial cost	(10 000)	(10 000)	(10 000)
Year 1 projected cash receipts	5 000	2 000	3 000
Year 2 projected cash receipts	5 000	4 000	3 000
Year 3 projected cash receipts	1 000	4 000	3 000
Year 4 projected cash receipts	nil	4 000	3 000
Total projected cash receipts			
Profit over four years			
Average annual profit			
Average rate of return			

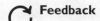 **Feedback**

Table 19.4 The ARR for Projects A, B and C (solution)

	Project A ($)	Project B ($)	Project C ($)
Initial cost	(10 000)	(10 000)	(10 000)
Year 1 projected cash receipts	5 000	2 000	3 000
Year 2 projected cash receipts	5 000	4 000	3 000
Year 3 projected cash receipts	1 000	4 000	3 000
Year 4 projected cash receipts	nil	4 000	3 000
Total projected cash receipts	**11 000**	**14 000**	**12 000**
Profit over four years	1 000	4 000	2 000
Average annual profit	250	1 000	500
Average rate of return	**2.5%**	**10%**	**5%**

Did you notice how this changes the situation? The project with the shortest payback period (Project A) actually has the lowest ARR.

Discounted cash flow – net present value

The result of the calculation in Activity 19.2 is not surprising since both methods entail different attitudes towards the time value of the investment. The payback method assumes that the fastest return should be preferred while the ARR looks at the average return over the investment period. However, neither method takes account of time preferences people have in comparing returns over time. Assume somebody owes you money. Would you prefer to receive the amount next week or in one year's time? Clearly the value of the money is not the same, for you would probably prefer the amount to be given back sooner rather than later. Similarly, if two equal amounts are invested with the same ARR, one over five years, the other over ten years, you would prefer the one which repays faster. The reason is that this amount could be invested elsewhere and yield even higher returns than you would achieve by tying up the capital over ten years. The method that has been developed to adjust payments or receipts that occur at different time periods is called *discounting*. Based on the concept of opportunity costs it takes account of investing the amount in alternative ways and allows the future returns of the investment be compared to its present value. The discount rate, the percentage by which future returns are adjusted to consider the underlying time preferences, is usually set at around the current rate of interest.

Present value tables (Table 19.5) are used to find the present value of anticipated future returns. It can be seen from Table 19.5 that the present value of $100 in four years' time discounted at a rate of 10 per cent is $0.683 \times 100 = \$68.30$.

Table 19.5 Extract from discount tables

Year	Present value (rate of discount 10%)
0	1.00
1	0.909
2	0.826
3	0.751
4	0.683
5	0.621

Present value of a stream of income over a number of years

If you are expecting an investment to yield a regular stream of income, you add the present values of the income for each of the years respectively.

Net present value

To calculate the estimated profit from an investment, subtract the initial outlay or cost from the present value as calculated above, to arrive at the *net present value (NPV)*. For example, a project involves an initial capital outlay of $350,000 and projected returns over four years are $100,000 in years 1 and 2 and $120,000 in years 3 and 4. The present value of the returns is calculated as follows. Using information from Table 19.5, the present value of $100,000 at the end of years 1 and 2 and $120,000 at the end of years 3 and 4 is shown in Table 19.6. The present value of the returns ($345,580) is actually less than the initial capital outlay, giving a (negative) NPV of $4420, so it is probably not worth considering the project.

Table 19.6 Present value calculations

Year 1	100 000 × 0.909	$90 900
Year 2	100 000 × 0.826	$82 600
Year 3	120 000 × 0.751	$90 120
Year 4	120 000 × 0.683	$81 960
Total		**$345 580**
Initial outlay		$350 000
NPV		**($4 420)**

The main advantage that NPV has over the other methods is that it takes account of the time value of money. However, neither interest rates nor cash flows can be estimated with absolute certainty, so there is an amount of guesswork that goes into these calculations.

Discounted cash flow – internal rate of return

Closely related to net present value, the *internal rate of return (IRR)* allows the user to work out the average rate of return on an investment throughout its lifetime. It concentrates on percentage returns on investment rather than on cash sums. IRR is that discount rate at which NPV = zero. Working through the following example and the activities that follow will show you how the IRR is calculated.

Consider Project X costing $200,000 with an income and present value (PV) as shown in Table 19.7. At a discount rate of 10 per cent the NPV of Project X is $323,920 − $200,000 = $123,920.

Table 19.7 Project X – earnings

Year	Earnings ($)	PV at 10% ($)
1	100 000	90 900
2	110 000	90 860
3	100 000	75 100
4	80 000	54 640
5	20 000	12 420
		323 920
Original outlay		200 000
NPV		**123 920**

 Activity 19.3

Now use the discounted cash flow tables in Appendix 2 to calculate the NPV at 30 per cent and 40 per cent.

Table 19.8 Project X – earnings and NPV at 10%, 30% and 40%

Year	Earnings ($)	PV at 10% ($)	PV at 30% ($)	PV at 40% ($)
1	100 000	90 900		
2	110 000	90 860		
3	100 000	75 100		
4	80 000	54 640		
5	20 000	12 420		
		323 920		
Original outlay		200 000	200 000	200 000
NPV		**123 920**		

Feedback

Table 19.9 Project X – NPV at 10%, 30% and 40% (solution)

Year	Earnings ($)	PV at 10% ($)	PV at 30% ($)	PV at 40% ($)
1	100 000	90 900	76 900	71 400
2	110 000	90 860	65 120	56 100
3	100 000	75 100	45 500	36 400
4	80 000	54 640	28 000	20 800
5	20 000	12 420	5 380	3 720
		323 920	**220 900**	**188 420**
Original outlay		200 000	200 000	200 000
NPV		**123 920**	**20 900**	**(11 580)**

From Table 19.9 you can see that the NPV at 30 per cent is $20,900, and at 40 per cent the NPV should be ($11,580) – i.e. a negative value. If you did not arrive at these figures go back over your calculations.

The IRR is that rate at which NPV is zero so in this case it lies between 30 and 40 per cent. To work out the exact rate:

1 Take the lower rate (30 per cent).

2 Add it to the difference between the two discount rates (10 per cent) multiplied by (the NPV at the lower rate divided by the sum of the two NPVs):

$$30 + 10 \times \frac{20{,}900}{(20{,}900 + 11{,}580)} = 36.4\%$$

Advantages and limitations of the IRR

The IRR enables a comparison with other rates of return on investment. However, because it concentrates on return, focusing on IRR exclusively ignores the actual value in monetary terms of the return on investment. Therefore, the NPV should always be considered as well. If the NPV is positive, the project should be accepted; if negative, it should be rejected. Also, the interpretation of the IRR can be misleading if the original outlay is not considered. An IRR of 10 per cent on a large capital outlay could be a better investment than an IRR of 15 per cent on a smaller capital sum.

Finally, as with all the other techniques discussed here, its accuracy depends on the accuracy of the forecasts, particularly on the amounts and timings of the anticipated cash flows. Different scenarios should be calculated to take into consideration changes in key conditions.

But regardless of the appraisal method, the most fundamental question is whether the investment is viable at all. At least there should be reasonable grounds for assuming that the investment will yield returns in the expected way. It is a general experience that often the figures are based on over-optimistic assumptions, particularly when a project is designed to attract support from decision-makers or investors. So whether a project is worthwhile is not decided by the figures alone but even more through the managerial judgement and intuition necessary for a critical assessment of the risks involved.

Assessment of affordability and sustainability of the investment

Viability, prudence, sustainability and affordability of capital investments should be seen in context (CIPFA 2002):

1   Capital investments should fit in with the overall financial planning of the organization. The forecast should include both capital and revenue expenditure because changes in revenue spending may change the scope for capital investments and vice versa. If staff expenditure is expected to increase over the following years because more doctors and nurses are needed, this should be considered in the assessment.

2   The direct effects of the capital investment on revenue expenditure should be analysed carefully: while capital investments are usually meant to increase productivity and to reduce staff and maintenance costs, they can have the opposite effect, particularly when standards are raised or new technology is used. For example, a higher proportion of single-bedded rooms makes a ward more expensive to operate because of the need for more nurses and higher cleaning costs. Likewise, the use of a new imaging device may add to staff and maintenance costs. The additional revenue required should be estimated and offset against any increase in income and/or against savings of running costs, which can be achieved through the capital investment.

3   The cash flow implications of the capital programme should be assessed to determine whether the organization is able to use its own funds or needs to take out an external loan to cover the cash requirements of the investment. If borrowing is required, you would assess whether the organization can afford to pay the interest even in the event of unfavourable economic circumstances. The principle of prudence requires that you also consider the impact of the loan on the balance sheet, particularly on the overall debt burden, to ensure sustainability of the organization in the future ('going concern').

4   In the public sector, capital investment programmes are governed by regulations. The proportion of public debt must be held at a stable level in relation to national income. As a rule of prudence, public organizations should only borrow to invest and not to fund current expenditure. Therefore, the capital programmes at different levels of the public health sector must be in line with overall government spending targets while ensuring that the annual rates for repayment and interest are realistic and affordable.

5   Partnerships between the public and private sector are increasingly common in the health sector. For example, private investors build new facilities and rent them back to the public sector. While this helps to keep the public capital budget down, a benefit for government is only achieved if the long-run costs of the scheme are less than they would have been had the public sector itself undertaken the project. Here again, in accordance with the principle of prudence, government should ensure that the benefits of any public-private partnership outweigh its cost.

Summary

Investment appraisal techniques are used to assist in capital investment appraisal when a full evaluation is not undertaken. These techniques are designed to analyse the return on the investment. They are all based on the initial capital outlay and the projected returns. The payback method looks only at the length of time it will take to recover the capital invested. The ARR takes account of the average annual rate of return on the investment. More sophisticated methods which use discounted cash flow techniques are the NPV, which depends both on an accurate forecast of returns and on the selection of an appropriate discount rate, and the IRR, which determines the discount rate at which the NPV is equal to zero. The principle of prudence aims to ensure that capital investments are affordable and sustainable and that option appraisal techniques are used in an appropriate way to ensure value for money.

Reference

CIPFA (2002) *The Role that Depreciation could Play in Local Government Finance*. London: CIPFA.

20 Financial issues in project management

Overview

Project management means taking a systematic approach to any undertaking within an organization which is not part of the routine work and has a defined beginning and end. In this chapter you will explore the implications this has for financial management and learn more about the different approaches and techniques to planning and monitoring activity and costs.

Learning objectives

By the end of this chapter you will be able to:

- outline the main stages and skills of project management
- describe principles of managing scope time, activity and costs in a project
- explain the earned value method

Key terms

Critical path analysis (CPA) A technique for analysing the time constraints of a project by identifying critical and non-critical tasks.

Earned value A method comparing the amount of projected work with what was actually accomplished to determine whether the project's cost and schedule performance is as planned.

Gantt chart A visual representation of the activities and the time required for implementing a project.

Logical framework A planning approach reflecting the logical structure of a project's objectives, activities and results. It summarizes what the project intends to do, how results will be monitored and evaluated and an assessment of risk.

Optimism bias The tendency for managers or stakeholders to be over-optimistic about key project parameters.

Project management A systematic approach to coordinating project inputs and processes in such a way that the desired outcomes are achieved.

What is project management?

As a manager you have to deal with projects in many different contexts. A key aspect is controlling costs but the planning of income and expenditure, the scheduling of activity and the closure of a project are also tasks that involve financial skills. However, project management should not be seen as an isolated activity focusing on costs, rather it includes a systematic approach to organization, leadership, team-building and conflict management as well as planning, decision-making and controlling the activities necessary to achieve the project goals.

- *A project* is a task with defined aims and objectives and which has a beginning and an end. This can be any form of undertaking such as a new building for a hospital, introducing IT, conducting a health promotion campaign or training programme for health workers, or any other finite task.
- *Project management* is the systematic approach to coordinating project inputs and processes in such a way that the desired outcomes are achieved. The project manager has to ensure that the objectives are met and that best use is made of time and resources.

Standardized approaches to project management

It is not uncommon to use a standardized approach to project management, if the undertaking has a large scope, a high level of complexity or involves many people. Standards are set rules and guidelines which have been approved by a recognized professional body. For example, the European system of quality standards is EN29000. If you want to know more about a special standard that is used in your country you may refer to professional organizations, government agencies or examine the website of the organization which has approved of the standard. Standards make projects comparable across organizations and ensure that the desired outcomes are achieved. Standardized management approaches are widely used, nationally and internationally. For example, to ensure that all their consultants use similar resources and work to the same standards of quality, consultancy firms may use standardized procedures for their many different projects.

Stages of project management

Even if you do not use a standardized approach, a clear structure of the project is important for various reasons:

- to reduce the risk of failure;
- to consider alternatives;
- to divide the workload between team members.

Typically, any project evolves over the following steps:

1 *Finding ideas and structuring problems:* making the project idea transparent and building a shared vision of what the project is about are among the first steps to

be taken. A common reason for project failure is lack of planning and lack of clarity of the project idea.

2 *Developing the project team and involving stakeholders:* the selection and development of a project team ensures that people with the right skills, experience and knowledge are in place. It is also useful to assess all direct responsibilities and expectations of stakeholders in order to ensure their support.

3 *Planning the project:* as a next step, an overall project plan is produced for the approval of all participants and stakeholders. The master plan is translated in a detailed plan for scheduling activity and budgeting costs.

4 *Implementing the project:* during implementation, careful monitoring and control of activity and costs is required.

5 *Evaluating and closing the project:* at the closure of the project a careful review of the management process and of the results is undertaken to evaluate the project and to learn lessons for the future.

Skills and knowledge areas for project management

Managing a project throughout its entire life cycle requires a range of skills which tie in with the specific financial management skills required. These skills complement each other and form the basis of project management (PMI Standards Committee 1999):

1 *Integration management* ensures that the different parts of the project fit together and that the relation of the project to the rest of the organization's activities is clearly defined.

2 *Scope management* ensures that all necessary activities are carried out and neither more nor less is done. So you would ensure that the project stays within its boundaries.

3 *Time management* ensures that all deadlines are kept and the project is completed within the planned time frame.

4 *Cost management* involves planning and monitoring of resources to ensure that the project stays within the budget limits.

5 *Quality management* ensures that the project meets its stated objectives. It involves in-built measures of quality assurance to eliminate undesirable performance failures.

6 *Human resource management* ensures that effective use is being made of the staff involved in the project in both staff selection and team development.

7 *Communications management* involves generation, collection and dissemination of information that is relevant for the project to be successful.

8 *Risk management* involves dealing systematically with the uncertainty around project implementation. It includes risk identification and quantification as well as risk response development and control (how to respond to threats and how to respond to changes in risk).

As a successful project manager you will need to have skills and competencies in all these areas. Many of these abilities are not generally different from other management roles. However, there is a range of methods and tools which are particularly suited to project management.

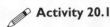
Activity 20.1

Think of a project that has recently been conducted in your organization.

1 How were the different skills represented in the project team?
2 In which ways were the different skills important for financial management of the project?

Feedback

1 It is clearly a role of leadership to keep the different activities of a project team together. Project teams are normally composed in a way that ensures all the relevant skills for managing the project are represented. For larger projects, such as building a new hospital, the organization may engage external cost engineers or quantity surveyors who monitor the project.

2 You may have found that managing risk, time and scope is closely integrated with financial management of the project, but all other activities also play an important role in cost control. For example, additional costs may arise due to poor communication within the project or a project may even fail if conflict within the team or with stakeholders is not resolved.

Planning a project

Any project needs to have a clear blueprint of its goals and objectives and associated control mechanisms. A comprehensive planning technique that is widely used in bi-lateral and multi-lateral health development programmes is the *logical framework*. The logical framework is not just a description of the project. Rather, it reflects the logical structure of the relationship between its objectives, activities and results, and specifies how to verify whether these objectives have been achieved. It also includes an assessment of risk indicating what assumptions outside the control of a project may influence its success. The central document is a plan which displays:

- goal;
- purpose;
- outputs;
- activity clusters per output.

For each of these categories measurable targets (indicators) and the means of their verification are identified. The overall plan provides a concise document to inform stakeholders. It can also serve in informing decision-making as it provides a clear visualization of risks and assumptions. A weakness of the method is that information for target verification may be lacking or of poor quality and it may be difficult to identify appropriate indicators for situations that are difficult to measure.

Controlling risk

The project manager should make provisions to ensure that financial risks are identified as early as possible. There are several ways of reducing risk or at least mitigating its impact on project performance. For example, before irreversible financial decisions are made, the costs and consequences of alternative options should be evaluated in order to enable informed choices. In complex projects, pilot studies may help to identify critical issues and to avoid adverse results, as valuable experience will be gained before the main project starts. Other approaches to risk control are related to contracting and insurance. Large projects, such as building a new hospital, bear a high financial risk due to unexpected events, which can be reduced by taking out insurance. Where contractors are hired for specific tasks or services are sourced out, the financial risk should be shared in a fair way between the contracting parties.

A particular pitfall in project management is the risk arising from *optimism bias*. This is the tendency for managers or stakeholders to be over-optimistic about key project parameters. Optimism bias may lead to adverse effects, such as under-estimation of capital costs and work duration or overestimation of the benefits of the project. The project team should address these issues in a systematic way by analysing the scope and objectives of the project. Project costs and work duration estimates should be based on empirical evidence from similar projects or past projects that have been implemented successfully. The evaluation of financial risk should also answer the questions of by how much costs could increase, work be delayed, or expected benefits be reduced for the project to remain worthwhile. Additional confidence can be gained if the project design is reviewed by an independent expert. Effective control systems should be in place to ensure that schedules and budgets are adhered to and risks that might arise during any phase of the project are controlled.

Planning the project budget

If external funding is required, funding opportunities should be identified at an early stage. Funding agencies usually require a statement of capacity including the applicant's most recent annual report and accounts to prove that the institution has a stable financial position and sufficient experience and resources to implement the project.

Planning a project budget is not different from planning any other budget, with the exception that a project is a separate financial entity requiring that its resources are identified, acquired, organized and combined for the specific purpose of the project (Pettinger 1997).

In practical terms, for each of the activities the associated resources are identified – for example, staff time, equipment, travel, accommodation, daily allowances etc.

Then the associated costs are calculated or estimated if correct information is not available. Preferably the zero-based budgeting approach should be used. Because project budgets are not part of the daily routine, a careful assessment of all financial risks is necessary. The budget should consider contingencies and build in an allowance to cover for unexpected expenditure which may arise during project implementation. Overheads are usually assigned to the budget, if they can be recovered from agencies funding the project.

The budget should clearly display the sources of funding and be accompanied by a document which explains and justifies each item.

Scheduling the project

Once you have arranged all tasks in a logical sequence you schedule the project by attaching time estimates, either beginning from the starting point or working backwards from the finishing date.

There are various methods for scheduling and visualizing activity, for example the *Gantt chart* and the *critical path method*.

- *A Gantt chart* provides a visual representation of the activities and the time required. The chart has a tabulated listing of the required activities and a graphic display with a separate bar for each activity, with the length of the bar representing the total time involved for the activity, using a calendar timescale bar across the top. The Gantt chart can show milestones and represent different types of activity using different symbols and colours. Milestones are major events that are suitable to monitor progress of the project.
- *A critical path chart* gives additional information on the overall time constraints of the project. This technique allows you to enter the earliest and the latest starting and finishing time for each task to calculate the float (the spare time) you have. From this you can see whether a task is critical, which means that a delay in the task causes a delay in the entire project, or non-critical, which means that some delay in the task does not endanger the timeliness of the entire project. The critical path method helps identify the fastest way of finishing a project and how to use spare time efficiently for non-critical tasks.

Activity 20.2

Suppose you have been asked to organize a fieldwork project that involves taking blood samples from people living in a remote area. Put the project activities in Table 20.1 in a logical sequence and display them in a Gantt chart. Note that some tasks can be performed simultaneously until the collection of samples starts.

Table 20.1 Project activities

Task	Duration in days
Arrange staff transport and accommodation	5
Analyse blood samples	5
Inform participants	7
Arrange for laboratory supplies and equipment	5
Train staff	10
Identify district for project	5
Collect blood samples	5
Select staff	4

↻ **Feedback**

Your Gantt chart should look similar to Figure 20.1.

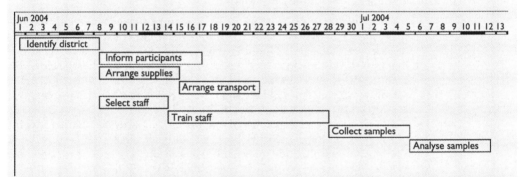

Figure 20.1 Gantt chart for blood sample field project

The Gantt chart provides a graphic representation of the duration of each task and shows parallel and overlapping tasks. The corresponding critical path chart would look similar to that shown in Figure 20.2.

The critical path is highlighted by arrows. This method provides more detail on the dependencies between tasks and gives more information as to whether the overall project will be completed on time by showing which activities are on the critical path and the float of non-critical tasks.

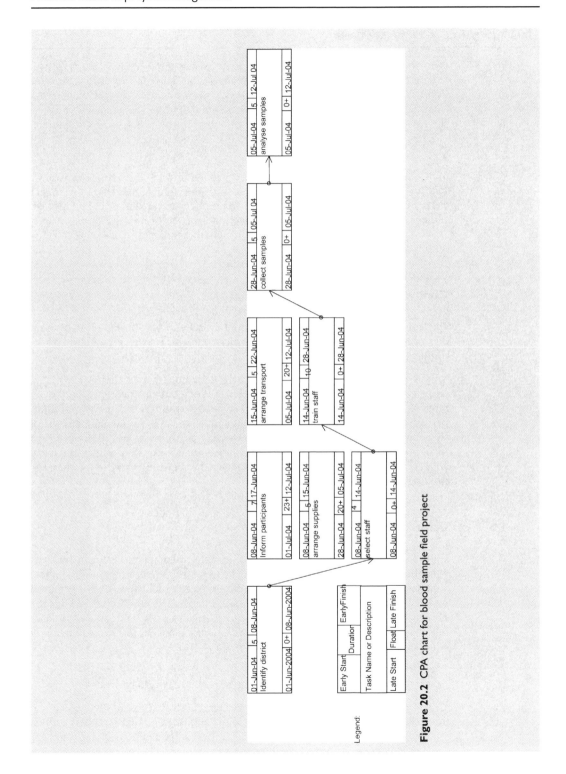

Figure 20.2 CPA chart for blood sample field project

Monitoring time, activity and costs

Once the detailed project plan has been agreed, you will start with the implementation of the project and ensure that all objectives are met. As you cannot monitor every single activity, the focus should be on the key critical factors that have a major impact on the implementation of the project, for example, avoiding delays in critical tasks, changes in funding or a partner withdrawing from the project. Contingency plans should be in place, if planned events don't materialize (Lewis 1997).

Short status reports may help you assess how much time the different tasks actually take and what progress has been made. Milestones are major events in a project that can be used to monitor progress and to produce intermediate reports for stakeholders and funding agencies. A milestone chart can easily be derived from a Gantt chart. It compares the scheduled and the actual completion dates of key events within the overall schedule.

Controlling costs

Controlling costs during the project is essential and several techniques can be used, depending on the complexity of the project and the reporting requirements of funding agencies.

A basic approach is a budget control chart which allows you to compare expected with actual expenditure. It gives you an account of what you have spent and what remains in the budget, and it helps you keep the overall balance as you may compensate budget items overspent with items underspent. A simple budget control sheet is sufficient when your institution is responsible for the accounting of income and expenditure of the project. In larger projects you may also need to keep an income and expenditure account that meets the accounting requirements of the funding institution.

Earned value

With a simple budget control chart you are able to compare the budgeted costs with those actually incurred. However, this does not tell you whether any budget variance is due to the activity being behind or ahead of schedule. This is achieved by a more sophisticated approach, the *earned value method*, which assesses both the dimension of variance to schedule and of variance to costs. The *schedule variance* tells you whether the project is ahead or behind the plan, the *cost variance* tells you whether the budget is over- or underspent.

The earned value method integrates both dimensions and allows the work in progress to be quantified. There are four measures you should be aware of:

1   The *budget at completion (BAC)*: this is the total budgeted cost of the project.
2   The *budgeted cost of the work scheduled (BCWS)*: the portion of costs that is equivalent to the portion of work that *should* be completed at a given time, for example, after one, two or three months. Because projects are not completed in

one step, the budget is broken down to the different phases of the project, according to the planned completion of each task.

3 The *budgeted cost of the work performed (BCWP)*: this is the portion of costs that is equivalent to the portion of work that has *actually* been completed at a given time. As work is completed it is considered *earned value*. The BCWP (actual) may differ from the BCWS (plan) because some tasks may take longer or shorter than planned and this variance is used to assess whether the project is on time.

4 The *actual cost of the work performed (ACWP)*: this can be in line with the budget or over- or underspent. Common reasons for differences between actuals and plan (the ACWP and the BCWP) are, for example, uncertainties of the budget estimates or price changes. ACWP is the cumulated cost incurred during a given period of time, as recorded by the accounting system.

Derived from these measures, variance is calculated as:

Schedule variance = BCWS – BCWP

Cost variance = BCWP – ACWP

Note that a negative variance means that more money was spent on the work accomplished than was planned. The cost variance can also be expressed as a ratio, the *cost performance index (CPI)*:

CPI = ACWP/BCWP

Activity 20.3

The following example illustrates the use of the earned value method. Suppose you are conducting a training project for health workers who are attending a course of one month's duration. The project has scheduled monthly costs of $20,000. The BAC is $200,000, so the project runs over ten months. Complete the three last rows in Table 20.2 by calculating the:

1 Schedule variance (BCWP – BCWS).
2 Cost variance (BCWP – ACWP).
3 Cost performance index (CPI = ACWP/BCWP).

Table 20.2 Training project for health workers – earned value schedule

Month	Scheduled budget (BCWS)	Earned value (BCWP)	Actual cost (ACWP)	Schedule variance	Cost variance	CPI
1	20	20	23			
2	40	30	35			
3	60	60	62			
4	80	90	87			
5	100	100	102			
6	120	130	135			
7	140	130	145			
8	160	160	165			
9	180	180	188			
10	200	200	231			

Feedback

As Table 20.3 shows, the planned training is behind schedule in months 2 and 7 (the schedule variance is negative) and ahead of schedule in months 4 and 6. Most of the time the budget is overspent, only in month 4 are the actual costs below the BCWP. The CPI shows this trend as a percentage.

Table 20.3 Training project for health workers – completed Earned value schedule

Month	Scheduled budget (BCWS)	Earned value (BCWP)	Actual cost (ACWP)	Schedule variance	Cost variance	CPI
1	20	20	23	0	−3	1.15
2	40	30	35	−10	−5	1.17
3	60	60	62	0	−2	1.03
4	80	90	87	10	3	0.97
5	100	100	102	0	−2	1.02
6	120	130	135	10	−5	1.04
7	140	130	145	−10	−15	1.12
8	160	160	165	0	−5	1.03
9	180	180	188	0	−8	1.04
10	200	200	231	0	−31	1.16

The idea behind these measures is that you can assess cost trends and forecast the estimated cost at completion (EAC). The case is simple when the actual costs are in line with the budgeted cost of the work scheduled. Then the EAC is the actual cost to date plus the remaining budget. If actual costs to date are higher than expected then there are two possibilities: you can either adjust the EAC by a percentage factor (the PCI) which takes account of the trend. Or if conditions have changed or if your first estimates of costs were flawed you need to recalculate the remaining budget based on new assumptions. In both cases you would have to plan cost cuts or get additional funding and you would also inform the relevant stakeholders about the cost performance of the project.

Table 20.4 shows a scenario where the work is ahead of schedule and the budget overspent.

Table 20.4 Earned value report showing work ahead of schedule and budget overspent

Task	Cumulative cost at 30 June			Variance		At completion 31 December		
Code	BCWS	BCWP	ACWP	Schedule	Cost	BAC	EAC	Variance
A4	550	600	680	50	−80	3 300	4 000	−700

Activity 20.4

The figures in Table 20.5 are taken from an earned value report. Are the tasks ahead or behind schedule? Is the budget over- or underspent? What is the forecast at completion?

Table 20.5 Extract from an earned value report

Task	Cumulative cost at 30 June			Variance		At completion 31 December		
Code	BCWS	BCWP	ACWP	Schedule	Cost	BAC	EAC	Variance
A4	550	600	680	50	−80	3 300	3 100	200
B1	300	250	200	−50	50	1 500	1 900	−400

 Feedback

Task A4 is ahead of schedule and overspent but the EAC will stay within the budget limits. Task B1 is behind schedule and underspent but a deficit is likely to occur at completion.

Cash flow analysis

Suppose the training project generates income in the form of fees which are paid by the course participants. You could then analyse the cash flow at the end of each month and assess whether income and expenditure targets have been met. Cash flow analysis only makes sense when there is an income during the duration of the project which is being used to cover project expenses. Cash flow is usually negative at the start of a project when fixed costs are high. If there is a steady income then costs may be recovered gradually. If, for example, income is obtained in separate quarterly or annual amounts, then a surplus (positive cash flow) may occur at the beginning of each period which is then compensated by the costs.

Evaluating and closing a project

While a continuing project evaluation during implementation has the advantage of reviewing timelines and enabling swift reactions, the additional post-project evaluation is absolutely necessary because you then have complete information on the entire management process, to derive lessons to be learned and to make conclusions on the final outcomes of the project.

The tasks to be performed at the end of a project should not be underestimated. A particular risk may arise from project drift. This is the phenomenon of declining commitment and performance at the end of a project arising from team members leaving the project for other jobs. Therefore, clear criteria for project closure should be set. These are also important for financial management because clear responsibilities and rules for financing of any unfinished work should be agreed. Finally, the project accounts must feed into and reconcile with the financial reporting system of the organization. Another important reason is that funding agencies set clear criteria for project closure.

1 Normally the last instalment of a grant is paid only after the project has ended and the final accounts are presented. Note that the bottom line of the actual project costs can be different from the BAC and EAC.
2 Many external funding agencies such as the EU have the additional requirement that for larger grants the final balance is only paid if an external audit report is produced by an approved auditor. Provisions for the time and costs of this should be made.

Summary

Project management is the systematic approach to coordinating project inputs and processes in such a way that the desired outcomes are achieved. The project manager has to ensure that the objectives are met and that best use is made of time and resources. A structured approach to project management helps to reduce the risk of failure, to consider all alternatives and to distribute the workload between team members appropriately. Various methods can be used for planning and scheduling activity and resources. During the implementation phase the monitoring system should focus on critical factors and allow for a timely response in taking corrective action. The earned value method can be used to forecast cost at completion and to ensure that the project stays within the budget limits. If the project generates a regular income, cash flow statements are a useful tool in assessing cost performance.

References

Lewis, J.P. (1997) *Fundamentals of Project Management*. New York: AMACOM.
Pettinger, R. (1997) *Introduction to Management*, 2nd edn. London: Macmillan.
PMI Standards Committee (1999) *A Guide to the Project Management Body of Knowledge*. Newton Square, USA: The Project Management Institute.

Appendix I

SOMEPLACE HOSPITAL Ltd

SPECIMEN ANNUAL ACCOUNTS
for the financial year ending 31 March 2004

Note that these accounts are not intended to represent the actual accounts of any particular hospital. They have been prepared to reflect, in general terms, the layout and presentation of the financial statements as discussed in Chapters 10 to 12.

Only those notes to the accounts which are relevant to the activities in this book are included.

Income Statement for the year ended 31 March 2004

	Note	2003/4 $000	2002/3 $000
Income from activities:			
Income from healthcare activities	3	**62,417**	55,070
Other operating income:			
Continuing operations	4	**5,363**	4,617
Operating expenses:			
Continuing operations	5–7	**(66,769)**	(58,458)
OPERATING PROFIT (LOSS)			
Continuing operations		**1,011**	1,229
Profit (loss) on disposal of fixed assets	8	**(143)**	(34)
PROFIT (LOSS) BEFORE INTEREST AND TAX		868	1,195
Interest receivable		**140**	152
Interest payable		**0**	0
Other finance costs		**0**	(32)
Corporation Tax		**(302)**	(395)
PROFIT (LOSS) FOR THE FINANCIAL YEAR		706	920
Dividends payable		**(529)**	(733)
RETAINED PROFIT (LOSS) FOR THE YEAR		177	187

Statement of Total Recognized Gains and Losses for the year ended 31 March 2004

	2003/4 $000	2002/3 $000
Profit for the year before dividend payments	**706**	920
Unrealized surplus (deficit) on fixed asset revaluations/indexation	**1,551**	330
Additions (reductions) in 'other reserves'	**0**	0
Total recognized gains and losses in the financial year	**2,257**	1,250

Balance Sheet as 31 March 2004

	Note	31 Mar 2004 $000	31 Mar 2003 $000
FIXED ASSETS			
Intangible assets	10	**169**	117
Tangible assets	11	**10,721**	14,110
		10,890	14,227
CURRENT ASSETS			
Stocks and works in progress	12	**765**	626
Debtors	13	**14,597**	7,064
Cash at bank and in hand	18	**7,203**	4,714
		22,565	12,404
CREDITORS: Amounts falling due within one year	15	**(5,501)**	(8,520)
NET CURRENT ASSETS (LIABILITIES)		**17,064**	3,884
TOTAL ASSETS LESS CURRENT LIABILITIES		**27,954**	18,111
CREDITORS: Amounts falling due after one year	15	**(7,798)**	0
PROVISIONS FOR LIABILITIES AND CHARGES		**(615)**	(298)
TOTAL ASSETS EMPLOYED	16	**19,541**	17,813
FINANCED BY:			
Share capital	17	**11,220**	11,220
Revaluation reserve		**3,108**	1,557
Income and expenditure reserve		**5,213**	5,036
TOTAL EQUITY		**19,541**	17,813

Cash Flow Statement for the year ended 31 March 2004

	Note	2003/4 $000	2002/3 $000
OPERATING ACTIVITIES			
Net cash inflow (outflow) from operating activities	18	**127**	5,184
RETURNS ON INVESTMENT AND SERVICING OF FINANCE:			
Interest received		**140**	152
Net cash inflow (outflow) from returns on investment and servicing of finance		**140**	152
CAPITAL EXPENDITURE			
Payments to acquire tangible fixed assets		**(1,814)**	(3,250)
Receipts from sale of tangible fixed assets		**5,251**	39
Payments to acquire/receipts from sale of intangible assets		**(87)**	0
Net cash inflow (outflow) from capital expenditure		**3,350**	(3,211)
DIVIDENDS PAID		**(733)**	(112)
Net cash inflow (outflow) before financing		**2,884**	2,013
Corporation Tax paid		**(395)**	(411)
FINANCING			
Capital raised		**0**	633
Capital repaid		**0**	0
Loans received		**0**	0
Loans repaid		**0**	0
Other capital receipts		**0**	0
Net cash inflow (outflow) from financing		**0**	633
Increase (decrease) in cash		**2,489**	2,235

NOTES TO THE ACCOUNTS

I. Acounting policies
This is normally a full and detailed statement of the accounting guidance that has been followed and the policies adopted in constructing the accounts. However, for the purposes of this example, only the relevant items in the statement of accounting policies are included.

1.1 Accounting convention
These accounts have been prepared under the historical cost convention modified to account for the revaluation of fixed assets at their value to the business by reference to their current costs.

Acquisition and discontinued operations
Definitions of acquired and discontinued operations . . .

Income recognition
Income is accounted for applying the accruals convention. The main source of income for the Someplace Hospital is from government funding of health care services. Income is recognized in the period in which the services are provided. Where income is received for a specific activity which is to be delivered in the following financial year, that income is deferred.

1.2 Tangible fixed assets
Capitalization
Tangible assets are capitalized if they are capable of being used for a period which exceeds one year and they:

— individually have a cost of at least $5,000; or
— collectively have a cost of at least $5,000, where the assets are functionally interdependent, they had broadly simultaneous purchase dates, are anticipated to have simultaneous disposal dates and are under single managerial control; or
— form part of the initial setting-up cost of a new building, irrespective of their individual or collective cost.

Valuation
Tangible fixed assets are stated at historic cost less accumulated depreciation and any impairment to the asset. Any costs such as installation directly attributable to bringing them into working condition are included in the cost.

Depreciation, amortization and impairments
Tangible fixed assets are depreciated at rates calculated to write them down to estimated residual value on a straight-line basis over their estimated useful lives. No depreciation is provided on freehold land, assets in the course of construction and assets surplus to requirements.

Leaseholds are depreciated over the primary lease term.

Equipment is depreciated on cost evenly over the estimated life of the asset using the following lives.

Medical equipment and engineering plant and equipment – 5 to 15 years
Furniture – 10 years
Mainframe information technology installations – 8 years
Soft furnishings – 7 years
Office and information technology equipment – 5 years
Set-up costs in new buildings – 10 years
Vehicles are depreciated over 5 years.

1.3 Intangible fixed assets

Intangible assets are capitalized when they are capable of being used by the hospital for more than one year; they can be valued; and they have a cost of at least $5,000.

Purchased computer software licences are capitalized as intangible fixed assets where expenditure of at least $5,000 is incurred. They are amortized over the shorter of the term of the licence and their useful economic lives.

Further notes on accounting policies would relate to such items as:

leases, government grants, stocks and works in progress, pension costs, liquid resources.

2. Segmental analysis
This note has not been included; it would normally give details of the business segments in which the hospital operates. Most health service organizations operate in only one sector.

3. Income from activities

	2003/4 $000	2002/3 $000
Government	35,687	28,111
Insurance schemes	25,898	26,105
Private patients	664	736
Other	168	118
	62,417	55,070

4. Other operating income

	2003/4 $000	2002/3 $000
Education, training and research	2,307	2,031
Other income	3,056	2,586
	5,363	4,617

5. Operating expenses

	2003/4 $000	2002/3 $000
Services supplied by other health care organizations	211	335
Directors' costs	438	390
Staff costs	38,431	34,222
Supplies and services:		
clinical	8,620	8,278
general	245	251
Establishment	1,208	1,014
Transport	112	68
Premises	2,730	3,298
Bad debts	8	8
Depreciation and amortization	1,395	2,580
Audit fees	124	57
Other auditor's remuneration	0	40
Clinical negligence	529	155
New hospital development	10,751	5,991
Ambulance and patients' transport	396	383
Laboratory services	294	311
Nurses' continuing education	100	115
Special initiatives	854	504
Consultancy fees	284	404
Other	39	54
	66,769	58,458

Further notes under operating expenses may provide detail of such items as clinical negligence charges and operating leases.

6. Employee costs and numbers
Notes under this heading would include a breakdown of employee costs, average number of employees under specified categories and details of management costs.

7. Payment policy
Notes under a heading such as this would include compliance with adopted codes of practice for paying creditors.

8. Profit (loss) on disposal of fixed assets

	2003/4 $000	2002/3 $000
Profit on disposal of land and buildings	0	
Loss on disposal of land and buildings	0	
Profit on disposal of plant and equipment	17	
Loss on disposal of plant and equipment	(160)	(34)
	(143)	(34)

9. Interest payable
Details of interest payable on finance leases and other loans.

10. Intangible fixed assets

	Software licences $000
Gross cost at 1 April 2003	121
Additions – purchased	87
Gross cost at 31 March 2004	208
Accumulated amortization at 1 April 2003	4
Provided during the year	35
Accumulated amortization at 31 March 2004	39
Purchased at 1 April 2003	117
Total at 1 April 2003	117
Purchased at 31 March 2004	169
Total at 31 March 2004	169

11. Tangible fixed assets

	Land	Buildings	Assets under constr'n & paym'ts on account	Plant & machinery	Transport equipment	Information technology	Furniture & fittings	**Total**
	$000	$000	$000	$000	$000	$000	$000	$000
Cost or valuation at 1 April 2003	1,953	9,213	421	14,088	121	229	10	26,035
Additions: – purchased	0	1,305	266	81	0	162	0	1,814
Impairments	0	0	0	0	0	0	0	0
Transfers	0	228	(228)	0	0	0	0	0
Revaluation of land	1,551	0	0	0	0	0	0	1,551
Disposals	(3,280)	(3,790)	0	(1,799)	(58)	0	0	(8,927)
At 31 March 2004	224	6,956	459	12,370	63	391	10	20,473
Accumulated depreciation at 1 April 2003	0	2,913		8,832	30	144	6	11,925
Provided during the year	(114)	304		1,100	20	49	1	1,360
Impairments	0	0		0	0	0	0	0
Reversal of impairments	0	0		0	0	0	0	0
Disposals	0	(1,886)		(1,624)	(23)	0	0	(3,533)
Accumulated depreciation at 31 March 2004	(114)	1,331		8,308	27	193	7	9,752
Net book value at 1 April 2003	1,953	6,300	421	5,256	91	85	4	14,110
Net book value at 31 March 2004	338	5,625	459	4,062	36	198	3	10,721

12. Stocks and work in progress

Further detail of stocks would normally be included here.

13. Debtors

	31 Mar 2004 $000	31 Mar 2003 $000
Amounts falling due within one year:		
Health scheme debtors	330	1,832
Provision for irrecoverable debts	(171)	(176)
Other prepayments and accrued income	12,930	3,557
Other debtors	1,508	1,851
	14,597	7,064

14. Details of investments (if any) held

15. Creditors

	31 Mar 2004 $000	31 Mar 2003 $000
Amounts falling due within one year:		
Health scheme creditors	1,390	4,724
Other trade creditors	1,988	2,433
Tax and social security costs	(3)	697
Obligations under finance leases and hire purchase contracts	0	0
Other creditors	337	343
Accruals and deferred income	1,789	323
	5,501	8,520
Amounts falling due after more than one year:		
Other*	7,798	0
	13,299	8,520

* The hospital has taken out a fixed interest loan in order to finance the building of a new hospital wing due for completion in 2006.

16. Provisions for liabilities and charges

This note includes details of provision for items such as pensions and legal claims and of adjustments to the provisions. It may also include details of the expected timing of associated cash flows.

17. Movements on reserves

	Revaluation reserve	Income & expenditure reserve	Total
	$000	$000	$000
At 1 April 2003	1,557	5,036	6,593
Transfer from income statement		177	177
Revaluation of land	1,551		1,551
At 31 March 2004	3,108	5,213	8,321

18. Reconciliation of operating surplus to net cash flow from operating activities

	2003/4 $000	2002/3 $000
Total operating profit (loss)	1,011	1,229
Depreciation and amortization charge	1,395	2,580
(Increase)/decrease in stocks	(139)	(119)
(Increase)/decrease in debtors	(7,533)	5,321
Increase/(decrease) in creditors and provisions	5,393	(3,827)
Net cash inflow/(outflow) from operating activities	127	5,184

18.2 Reconciliation of net cash flow to movement in net debt

	2003/4 $000
Increase/(decrease) in cash in the period	2,489
Cash inflow (outflow) from (decrease)increase in liquid resources	0
Change in net debt resulting from cash flows	2,489
Non-cash changes in debt	0
Net debt at 1 April 2003	4,714
Net debt at 31 March 2004	7,203

18.3 Analysis of changes in net debt

	At 31 March 2004 $000	Cash changes in year $000	Non-cash changes in year $000	At 1 April 2003 $000
Cash at bank and in hand	7,203	2,489	0	4,714
Bank overdrafts	0	0	0	0
	7,203	2,489	0	4,714

Appendix 2

Discount table

Present value factors (present value of one unit)

Number of years	5%	10%	15%	Discount rate 20%	25%	30%	35%	40%
1	0.9524	0.9091	0.8696	0.8333	0.8000	0.7692	0.7407	0.7143
2	0.9070	0.8264	0.7561	0.6944	0.6400	0.5917	0.5487	0.5102
3	0.8638	0.7513	0.6575	0.5787	0.5120	0.4552	0.4064	0.3644
4	0.8227	0.6830	0.5718	0.4823	0.4096	0.3501	0.3011	0.2603
5	0.7835	0.6209	0.4972	0.4019	0.3277	0.2693	0.2230	0.1859
6	0.7462	0.5645	0.4323	0.3349	0.2621	0.2072	0.1652	0.1328
7	0.7107	0.5132	0.3759	0.2791	0.2097	0.1594	0.1224	0.0949
8	0.6768	0.4665	0.3269	0.2326	0.1678	0.1226	0.0906	0.0678
9	0.6446	0.4241	0.2843	0.1938	0.1342	0.0943	0.0671	0.0484
10	0.6139	0.3855	0.2472	0.1615	0.1074	0.0725	0.0497	0.0346
11	0.5847	0.3505	0.2149	0.1346	0.0859	0.0558	0.0368	0.0247
12	0.5568	0.3186	0.1869	0.1122	0.0687	0.0429	0.0273	0.0176
13	0.5303	0.2897	0.1625	0.0935	0.0550	0.0330	0.0202	0.0126
14	0.5051	0.2633	0.1413	0.0779	0.0440	0.0254	0.0150	0.0090
15	0.4810	0.2394	0.1229	0.0649	0.0352	0.0195	0.0111	0.0064
16	0.4581	0.2176	0.1069	0.0541	0.0281	0.0150	0.0082	0.0046
17	0.4363	0.1978	0.0929	0.0451	0.0225	0.0116	0.0061	0.0033
18	0.4155	0.1799	0.0808	0.0376	0.0180	0.0089	0.0045	0.0023
19	0.3957	0.1635	0.0703	0.0313	0.0144	0.0068	0.0033	0.0017
20	0.3769	0.1486	0.0611	0.0261	0.0115	0.0053	0.0025	0.0012

Glossary

Absorption costing A costing approach recovering the average cost of a service.

Accruals Expenses that the organization has incurred during the accounting period but for which invoices have not yet been received.

Accruals accounting An accounting system that recognizes revenue or costs as earned in the period when the transaction takes place (in contrast to cash accounting which only records transactions when cash is received or paid).

Asset Something that is owned by the organization; assets represent the *use* of organizational funds.

Asset turnover The amount of income generated for each unit invested in fixed assets: income/average fixed assets.

Audit trail A tool for checking data integrity allowing each transaction to be tracked down from the highest level of aggregation to the single entry of the feeder system and vice versa.

Average rate of return A measure of profitability, allowing investments with different capital outlays to be compared. The average rate of return is calculated as the ratio of the average cash inflow to the amount invested.

Balance sheet A statement of the total assets, liabilities and capital of an organization at a given moment.

Balanced budget strategy A strategy that ensures that the total of all expenditure budgets is equal to the total income budget.

Balanced scorecard A systematic approach to performance management, focusing not only on financial targets but also on customer needs, internal processes, learning and innovation.

Base rate The average cost across all DRGs. Base rates are not only calculated for individual hospitals but also to compare cost per case across a region or the entire country.

Beveridge system A health system funded through public revenue raised by general taxation, named after Sir William Beveridge.

Bismarck system A health system funded through payroll-based social health insurance contributions, named after Otto von Bismarck.

Bottom-up costing A detailed approach identifying the costs of all inputs.

Break-even activity level The activity level where total income equals total cost.

Budget A tool for relating planned resource consumption to a period of time.

Budget cycle The annual sequence of planning, budgeting, controlling and reporting to enable decisions on how an organization will use its resources.

Budget summarization hierarchy A budget structure reflecting the distribution of financial responsibility and accountability within large organizations. Single budget items of sub-units are combined to become totals of the next level in hierarchy.

Capital The funds invested in the organization by its owner or owners (accountancy definition).

Capital budgets Budgets that relate to items appearing in the balance sheet, such as the acquisition or disposal of property belonging to the organization.

Case-mix index A measure of disease severity across all cases treated in an entire department or hospital during a year, usually calculated as the sum of all relative costs weights divided by the number of cases.

Case-mix system An information system combining patient-related activity data with financial data on resource use.

Cash budgets (cash flow forecasts) Budgets which profile cash flows over the budget period, to ensure that there is enough cash to meet operational and other needs.

Cash flow forecast (cash budgets) Budgets which profile cash flows over the budget period, to ensure that there is enough cash to meet operational and other needs.

Cash flow statement A statement summarizing the inflows and outflows of cash over the accounting period.

Co-payments (user fees) Direct payments made by users of health services as a contribution to their cost (eg prescription charges).

Corporate governance Structures and functions describing the distribution of rights and responsibilities within an organization and the rules for decision-making among the different participants, such as the board, managers, owners or government.

Corruption Misuse of a position for dishonest gain, particularly the offering, giving, soliciting or acceptance of an inducement or reward, which may influence the action of the position-holder.

Cost allocation Charging an entire cost to the cost centre that is directly responsible for incurring it.

Cost apportionment Sharing a central cost between cost centres in proportion to the level of use each cost centre makes of it.

Cost centre Any activity or unit of organization for which you want to identify costs.

Cost profile A typical pattern of the costs associated with a category of patient or group of patients.

Cost variance A variance that arises because the cost of resources was greater or lower than anticipated.

Cost weight A factor reflecting the relative cost of a single diagnosis related group (DRG). By definition the cost weight of the base rate is 1.0, DRGs with a resource use below average have a cost weight < 1, above average of >1.

Critical path analysis A technique for analysing the time constraints of a project by identifying critical and non-critical tasks.

Current assets Short-term resources either held in the form of cash or expected to become cash within the next 12 months.

Current liabilities Amounts due for payment within 12 months from the balance sheet date.

Depreciation The process of accounting for the reduction in value of an asset over the period of its useful life.

Diagnosis related group (DRG) Classification system that assigns patients to categories on the basis of the likely cost of their episode of hospital care. Used as basis for determining level of prospective payment by purchaser.

Direct cost Resources used in the design, implementation, receipt and continuation of a health care intervention.

Discounted cash flow A method of comparing the profitability of alternative investments which takes the time value of money into account.

Discount rate The rate at which future costs and outcomes are discounted to account for time preference.

Discounting A method for adjusting the value of costs and outcomes which occur in different time periods into a common time period, usually the present.

Double entry book-keeping A system of record-keeping which recognizes that there are two sides to every transaction.

DRG creep (upcoding) A form of DRG misclassification leading to unjustified high reimbursement levels.

Earned value A method comparing the amount of projected work with what was actually accomplished to determine whether the project's cost and schedule performance is as planned.

Economy Purchasing resources at least cost.

Effectiveness The extent to which an intervention produces a beneficial result under usual conditions of clinical care.

Efficiency index A performance indicator combining the change of activity with the corresponding change of costs.

Efficiency variance A variance that arises because the labour input or the cost of overheads was higher or lower than planned.

Entity concept The unit for which the accounts are prepared; separate and distinct from its employees.

Feeder system The data input system of the financial reporting system responsible for recording and processing all financial transactions.

Financial accounting Financial information for external users reflecting the performance and financial standing of the organization.

Financial controls Systems to maintain probity at all levels of the organization through adherence to rules of governance, laws, financial regulations and internal policies.

Financial (budgetary) cost The accounting cost of a good or service usually representing the original (historical) amount paid, distinct from the opportunity cost.

Financial directions Rules and procedures describing the key financial responsibilities of the financial director and the chief executive officer.

Financial management Managerial activities of obtaining and disbursing funds, financial planning, reporting and risk management.

Financial reporting system An information system performing all aspects of the accounting process, involving the recording and processing of financial transactions as well as the producing of reports for various purposes.

Fixed assets Assets acquired for continuing use within the organization with a view to enabling it to carry out its normal operations.

Fixed costs A cost of production that does not vary with the level of content.

Flexible budget A budget showing comparative costs for a range of levels of activity.

Flexible budgeting Systems designed to allow budgets to respond to changes in workload and activity as the budget period progresses.

Fraud An intentional deception or misrepresentation that could result in some unfair gain. Financial fraud may involve activities such as forgery, falsification or alteration of documents as well as theft, destruction or misappropriation of funds, or misuse of facilities.

Gantt chart A visual representation of the activities, their sequence and the time required for implementing a project.

Gearing (leverage) Indicator of whether an organization can meet its long-term liabilities; gearing is calculated as interest-bearing debt/non-interest-bearing debt.

General ledger (nominal ledger) The main account book which consolidates the record of financial activities and allows the bottom line of net earnings to be calculated.

Going concern Assumes the entity will continue to exist into the foreseeable future, and there is no intention to close it down or make drastic operational cutbacks.

Hierarchy of control The combination of regulations and procedures to ensure openness, integrity and accountability in running an organization.

High-level controls Actions implemented at board level and above as part of the governance system, to ensure that budgetary controls and audit systems are in place.

Historic and current cost Historic cost reflects the original cost of an asset, current cost reflects the replacement cost.

Income statement (income and expenditure account) A summary of income and expenditure over the accounting period.

Incremental budgeting An approach which involves taking the previous period's budget and adjusting the figures to reflect the changes in planned activity levels and in costs and prices for the forthcoming year.

Indirect costs The value of resources expended by patients and their carers to enable individuals to receive an intervention.

Internal pricing Charging for services between units of the same organization with the aim of increasing cost-consciousness and efficiency.

Internal rate of return The discount rate where the net interest value is zero.

Job description A document defining the level of authority, responsibility and accountability of a job.

Lagging measures Historical indicators that inform on past performance.

Leading measures Future-directed indicators that a specific outcome is likely to be achieved.

Liability Something that is owed by the organization; liabilities represent the *source* of funds.

Liquidity (acid test) ratio A more critical test of an organization's ability to pay than the working capital ratio, the liquidity ratio excludes stock from the calculation, using cash + debtors/current liabilities.

Logical framework A planning approach reflecting the logical structure of a project's objectives, activities and results. It summarizes what the project intends to do, how results will be monitored and evaluated and an assessment of risk.

Long-term liabilities Amounts due for payment more than 12 months after the balance sheet date.

Low-level controls Activity specific to operational aspects of the organization, for example, separating duties to minimize the risk of fraud in the recording and authorizing of financial transactions.

Management accounting Information for internal users to help them run the organization such as budgets, plans, costings and financial appraisals of service developments.

Management reporting system The information system supporting the running of an organization. Management reports include both financial and non-financial information and can be produced for either strategic or operational purposes.

Marginal costing A costing approach recovering the variable cost of a service.

Marketing mix The mix of factors (price, product, place, promotion) to be controlled so that a service is provided in adequate quality and quantity.

Master budget The coordinated overall budget which combines the functional budgets, the capital budget and the cash flow budget with the budgeted income statement and balance sheet for the forthcoming period.

Materiality Those items that are significant enough to affect evaluation or decisions.

Money measurement Those items to which a monetary value can be attributed are included in the accounts.

Net book value (NBV) The historic or original cost of an asset minus accumulated depreciation to date.

Net present value The present value minus the initial capital outlay. If it is negative it is not worth pursuing the project.

New public management An approach to government involvement with the application to private sector management techniques.

Operational (technical, productive) efficiency Using only the minimum necessary resources to finance, purchase and deliver a particular activity or set of activities (ie avoiding waste)

Operating expenses The costs incurred by an organization in the course of its ordinary activities.

Operating income The income earned by an organization in the course of its ordinary activities.

Operating surplus (deficit) The difference between the operating income and operating expenses; a deficit will be incurred when expenses exceed income.

Opportunity (economic) cost The value of the next best alternative forgone as a result of the decision made.

Optimism bias The tendency for managers or stakeholders to be over-optimistic about key project parameters.

Outcomes Change in status as a result of the system processes (in the health services context, the change in health status as a result of care).

Overhead costs Costs that are not incurred directly from providing patient care but are necessary to support the organization overall (eg personnel functions).

Payback method An appraisal technique evaluating how long it will take to repay the initial investment.

Performance indicators Financial and non-financial measures used for monitoring activity levels, efficiency and quality of service provision by comparing actual with expected results.

Performance measures or ratios Techniques used to interpret financial statements.

Prepayments Payments made during the accounting period in respect of benefits which will be enjoyed in a future accounting period.

Present value The amount of money that a stream of cash inflows receivable in the future is currently worth. Future cash flows are multiplied by a defined discount factor to obtain the present value.

Private/public mix Mix of public and private funders and providers of health care.

Profiling The technique used to adjust for seasonal variations within a budget, so that actual progress can be monitored against the budget.

Profit margin (operating margin) A measure of profitability: operating profit/ surplus as a percentage of income.

Project management A systematic approach to coordinating project inputs and processes in such a way that the desired outcomes are achieved.

Prospective payment Paying providers before any care delivered based on predefined activity levels and anticipated cost.

Provider payment methods The different ways of paying health care providers such as fee-for-service, capitation and case base reimbursement.

Prudence (conservatism) A concept that requires all costs or losses to be recognized as soon as they are foreseen; not to record anticipated profits until actually realized.

Reducing balance method A method of depreciation which assumes the greatest reduction in the value of an asset will be in the earliest years of its useful economic life; each accounting period depreciation is calculated as a percentage of the asset's net book value at the beginning of the accounting period.

Regulation Government intervention to achieve specific objectives in the health sector through legal controls and incentives.

Reserves Funds theoretically due to the owners but which have been retained within the organization for some reason; the most common reserves are retained surplus or profit.

Residual claimant status The arrangements under which a person or agency – the residual claimant – is entitled to retain an organization's surplus or is held responsible to bear its financial loss.

Residual value The value at which an asset is considered likely to be sold at the end of its useful economic life.

Retained surplus (deficit) The surplus or deficit that remains after all expenses have been paid, interest payments on loans have been made and taxes and dividends, where applicable, have been paid.

Return on capital employed The return on capital invested in an organization calculated as profit before interest and tax/relevant net assets × 100.

Revenue budgets Budgets that relate to items in the operational activities of the organization.

Semi-variable costs Costs that contain both a fixed and a variable element.

Share capital Funds that have been invested in an organization by its shareholders.

Shareholders' funds The share capital and reserves of an organization.

Staff budgets Budgets that detail staff numbers at all levels and associated staff costs.

Stakeholder An individual or group with a substantive interest in an issue (ie interest group), including those with some role in making a decision or its execution.

Standing orders Rules that are permanently in force, outlining the general terms of managing the organization.

Stepped costs Costs that behave like fixed costs until certain thresholds are reached; when activity increases beyond each threshold, costs step to a higher level and remain fixed until the next threshold level of activity is reached.

Straight-line method A method of depreciation in which the estimated residual value is subtracted from the original cost of an asset and the depreciation is spread evenly over the useful economic life of that asset.

Target pricing A pricing approach adding a mark-up to the cost per unit of service in order to make a profit.

Top-down costing An approach based on average costs.

Treasury management Activities ensuring the organization has enough cash to meet all its financial obligations.

Trial balance A list of all the balances in an organization's book of account; this is usually the first step in preparing the annual accounts.

Unit of activity (currency) The unit used to measure activity, such as operations, bed-days or laboratory tests.

Usage variance A variance that arises because the volume of resources used was higher or lower than planned.

Useful economic life The period over which the owner of an asset will derive some economic benefit from its use.

Variable cost A cost of production that varies directly with the level of output.

Variance The difference between planned and actual activity.

Working capital (net current assets) Current assets minus current liabilities; this is the capital that is used in day-to-day operations.

Working capital cycle The cycle in which cash is used to pay creditors and also to pay staff and to purchase supplies, so enabling the organization to generate income from its operations which results either in immediate cash payments or in debtors who will, in due course, pay cash to settle their debts.

Working capital ratio (current ratio) A measure that compares current assets with current liabilities to analyse the organization's ability to meet its short-term obligations; it is calculated as current assets/current liabilities.

Zero-based budgeting A budgeting method that identifies and costs all of the inputs that will be required to achieve the desired level of activity and outcome.

Index

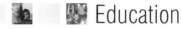
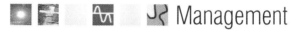
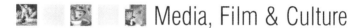
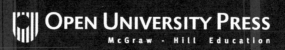